Biomedical Signal and Image Examination With Entropy-Based Techniques

Biomedical and Robotics Healthcare

Series Editors: Utku Kose, Jude Hemanth, Omer Deperlioglu

Biomedical Signal and Image Examination With Entropy-Based Techniques
Dr. V. Rajinikanth, Dr. K. Kamalanand, Dr. C. Emmanuel and Dr. B. Thayumanavan

For more information about this series, please visit: https://www.routledge.com/Biomedical-and-Robotics-Healthcare/book-series/BRHC

Biomedical Signal and Image Examination With Entropy-Based Techniques

Dr. V. Rajinikanth, Dr. K. Kamalanand,
Dr. C. Emmanuel and Dr. B. Thayumanavan

CRC Press
Taylor & Francis Group
Boca Raton London New York

CRC Press is an imprint of the
Taylor & Francis Group, an **informa** business

First edition published 2021
by CRC Press
6000 Broken Sound Parkway NW, Suite 300, Boca Raton, FL 33487-2742

and by CRC Press
2 Park Square, Milton Park, Abingdon, Oxon, OX14 4RN

ISBN: 978-0-367-47394-5 (hbk)
ISBN: 978-0-367-47724-0 (ebk)

Typeset in Times
by KnowledgeWorks Global Ltd.

Contents

Preface

Entropy is a measure of disorder or uncertainty associated with a system. Having its roots in the theory of thermodynamics, the concepts of entropy have branched to several domains including information theory. In recent years, the theory of entropy has made a significant breakthrough in the field of biomedical signal and image analysis leading to the development of computational algorithms for the mass screening of various diseases of the physiological systems. Entropy measures such as the Shannon's, Tsallis, Renyi, Kapur, etc, have been utilized for the examination of various biosignals and images by providing useful markers for various diseases.

Electrophysiology deals with the acquisition and analysis of the electrical signals associated with the physiological systems. The electrophysiological signals such as the Electrocardiograms (ECG), Electromyograms (EMG), Electroencephalograms (EEG), etc., and medical images such as X-ray images, Computed Tomography images, Magnetic Resonance Images, Ultrasound images, etc., have potential diagnostic information which needs to be identified using computerized algorithms for the mass screening of diseases. In this regard, the Entropy measures of electrophysiological signals and images serve as useful diagnostic markers for several diseases.

This book titled "Biomedical Signal and Image Examination with Entropy Based Techniques" presents the basics of entropy and the applications of entropy in the field of biomedical signals and image analysis.

The book is organized as follows:

Chapter 1 of this book presents a detailed introduction to the basics of entropy along with several entropy measures. This chapter also presents various techniques and methods for estimation of various entropy measures. Further, the concepts of chaos theory, the parameters involved in chaotic analysis and the relationship between chaotic measures and entropy is presented.

Chapter 2 presents the various types of biosignals, evaluation methods and instrumentation involved in their measurement. Further, the variation in entropy measures and other parameters utilized for chaos analysis is analyzed using suitable examples of biosignals acquired in normal and pathological conditions.

Chapter 3 presents the information regarding various medical imaging procedures widely considered in the hospitals and its thresholding using the Otsu and other related entropy techniques and its evaluation. This chapter also provides the choice of the various image modalities to evaluate a disease and also presents the traditional and computer based evaluation procedures with appropriate results attained with the MATLAB software.

Chapter 4 shows the entropy assisted image processing procedures using the gray-scale and the RGB scale medical images, and the result confirms that the Shannon's entropy offers better result. In this work, a case study on COVID-19 image examination is presented and discussed with appropriate results.

Chapter 5 depicts the appropriate results to confirm the eminence of the entropy-based thresholding. In this work the evaluation of the fundus retinal images, brain

MRI and the breast thermal imaging is discussed. The disease in eye, brain and the breast section is also examined using a chosen computerised examination technique.

The authors express their gratitude to the Editors, Dr. Utku Kose and Dr. Marc Gutierrez, CRC Press, for their continuous support. The authors thank Nick Mould, Editorial Assistant CRC press for his support. It was a pleasure working with them.

Dr. V. Rajinikanth
Dr. K. Kamalanand
Dr. C. Emmanuel
Dr. B. Thayumanavan

Author Biographies

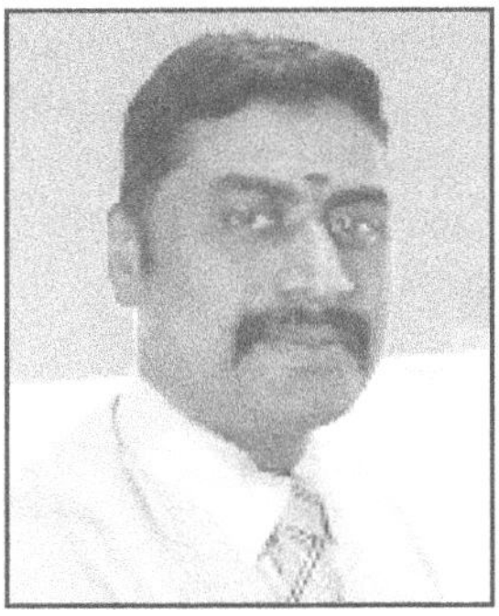

Dr. V. Rajinikanth is a Professor in the Department of Electronics and Instrumentation Engineering at St. Joseph's College of Engineering, Chennai, Tamil Nadu, India. He has recently edited books titled *Advances in Artificial Intelligence Systems*, Nova Science publisher, USA and *Applications of Bat Algorithm and its Variants*, Springer, Singapore. He is the Associate Editor of International Journal of Rough Sets and Data Analysis (IGI Global, US, DBLP, ACM dl) and is editing/has edited special issues for journals, such as *Current Signal Transduction Therapy*, *Current Medical Imaging Reviews* and *Open Neuroimaging Journal*. His main research interests include medical imaging, machine learning, and computer aided diagnosis, as well as data mining.

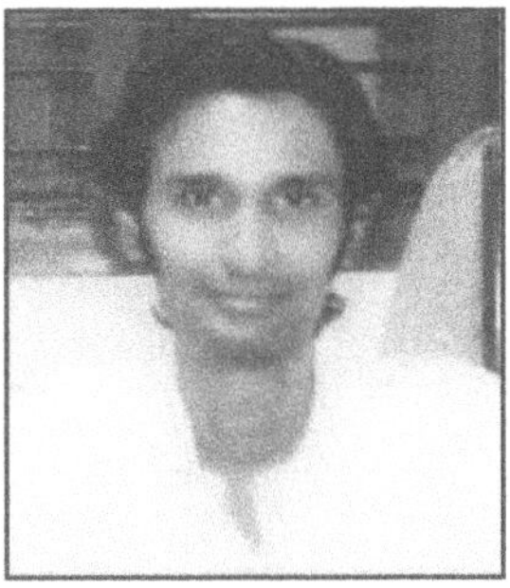

Dr. K. Kamalanand completed his Ph.D. at MIT Campus, Anna University in the field of intelligent modelling and analysis of HIV/AIDS infection. At present he is an Assistant Professor at the Department of Instrumentation Engineering, Madras Institute of Technology Campus, Anna University, Chennai, Tamil Nadu, India. He has co-authored and edited four text/reference books and has served as a Guest Editor for the *European Journal for Biomedical Informatics*, *Current Bioinformatics*, and *Current Signal Transduction Therapy*. He is a member of the Council of Asian Science Editors and is a Fellow at International Society of Biotechnology.

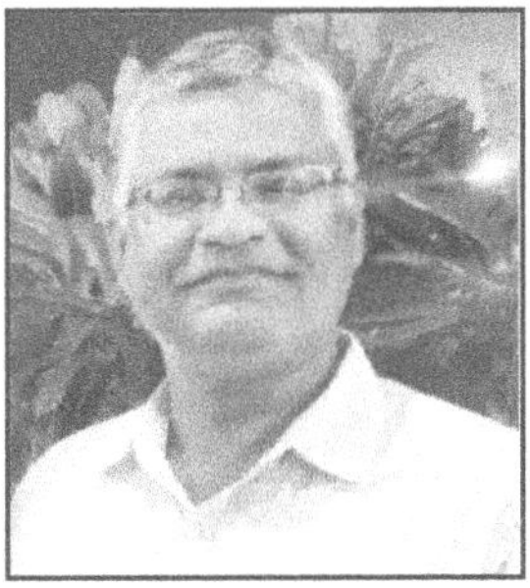

Dr. C. Emmanuel was born in Tiruchirappalli, Tamil Nadu. He is a Professor and Director of the Department of Academics & Research, Gleneagles Global Health City, Chennai, Tamil Nadu, India. Besides computational molecular medicine, his research interests include computer aided design and biomedical engineering. He is nationally renowned for his books, academic and scientific work, and has served as an editorial board member to various scientific journals. He has published several research articles and is a recipient of several awards and honors.

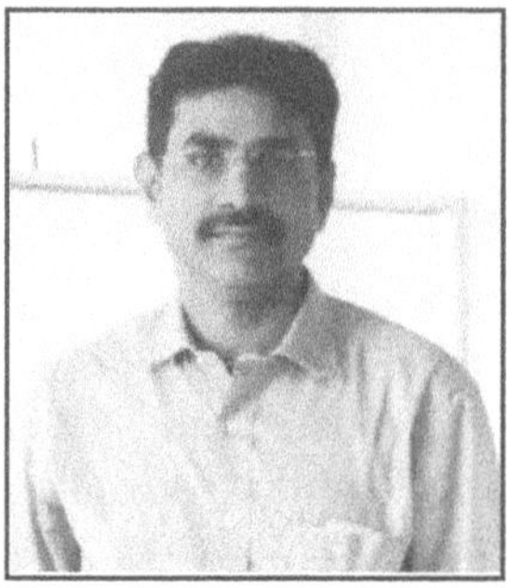

Dr. B. Thayumanavan received his M.D.S. from Tamil Nadu Government Dental College and his B.D.S. from Sree Balaji Dental College and Hospital, Chennai, Tamil Nadu India. At present he is a Professor and the Dean of Sathyabama University Dental College and Hospital, Chennai. He has a teaching experience of more than 16 years and has published several books and papers in international journals and conference proceedings. He has also supervised several dissertations, organized quite a few conferences and has chaired numerous scientific sessions too.

1 Introduction to Entropy and Chaos

Most of the physical and chemical processes can be investigated using the first and second laws of thermodynamics. These two laws are the most basic and fundamental for the analysis and understanding of the mechanisms involved in the functioning of such systems and processes. Biological systems and processes are a complex combination of physical and chemical processes and can efficiently be studied using the first and second laws of thermodynamics. Also, the third law of thermodynamics is of great importance in the analysis of such processes.

Several complex laws derived mathematically contributes to classic thermodynamics. However, the introduction of the concepts of statistical mechanics in the field of thermodynamics, gives rise to a new field namely, statistical thermodynamics. The aspects of statistical thermodynamics help in the identification of the actual or physical meaning of the parameters in the mathematical equations of classical thermodynamics.

The first law of thermodynamics deals with the law of conservation of energy and states that "a perpetual motion machine of the first kind is impossible". In other words, the first law states that energy can neither be created nor destroyed. While the first law deals with the energy of a system, the second law deals with another important quantity known as the 'entropy of a system'. The entropy of a system is a quantification of the disorder associated with a system or the randomness associated with a system (Martyushev & Seleznev, 2006; Kamalanand & Jawahar, 2018). In an irreversible process, the entropy is an ever-increasing function of time. At this point, it needs to be mentioned that the best example of an irreversible process is the biological life, from birth to death. Hence, biological systems are best described by the entropy associated with it and this particular parameter has proved itself to be an excellent descriptor of the microscopic and macroscopic processes associated with it (Brooks et al., 1989; Gladyshev, 1999; Wilson, 1968). Further, the analysis and quantification of energy and entropy associated with a biological system also provides information on the physiological and pathological states of the system. This book, in particular describes the applications of entropy analysis in the study of medical signals and images acquired from the human body. Since, the quantification of entropy in bio-signals and images has the potential to offer new biomarkers or parameters for the diagnosis and staging of several diseases of the human physiological system, such methods and techniques are described in detail.

The variations in entropy of processes are well associated with the increase in the disorder. An increase in entropy implies a loss of information since entropy and information are very closely related. A higher entropy is associated with more randomness, disorder, uncertainty and potential information, whereas, a lower entropy is associated with non-randomness, order, reliability, and stored information

(Kvålseth 2016). Hence a higher entropy relates to freedom whereas, a lower entropy relates to constraints (Daniel 2009).

1.1 PROBABILITY CALCULATIONS

Since the calculation of probability plays an important role in the estimation of entropy (Frank & Smith, 2010), this session describes certain basic mathematical definitions and techniques for the understanding of probability calculations.

Probability is an important aspect in entropy calculations and hence the randomization of the problem is required. In other words, entropy is closely related to the uncertainty involved (Maassen & Uffink, 1988). To explain probability, it requires the understanding of the statement "there occurs an event '*A*' for every realization of a set of conditions". For example, if a material is heated above its boiling point (which is the set of conditions involved), the material is converted into vapour state (which is the event '*A*'). A specific event that occurs for each and every realization of the set of conditions is known as a certain event. If the event does not occur, it is known as an impossible event and finally a random event is a case when the event may or may not occur. The probability of occurrence of the event A is given by $P(A)$ and is a value which quantitatively expresses the probability. This mathematical probability is a measure of the level of uncertainty or certainty involved in a process.

In the case of the quantification of the frequency of occurrence of an event, the statistical definition of probability can be obtained. In this case, the probability of an event A, given by $P(A)$ is equal to the number of possible outcomes in the favour of the event A divided by the number of all possible outcomes.

$$P(A) = \frac{f}{N}$$

where, f is the number or count of a particular event and N is the total number of trials. Thus, the probability $P(A)$ can be realized as a function of the event A, defined on the field of events (S).

$P(A)$ has the following properties:

- For every event A and field (S), $P(A) \geq 0$.
- For a certain event U, $P(U) = 1$

Following this, the concepts of statistical probability arises, which appears more realistic in the practical aspects of computation. In this field, the computation of probability requires a large number of trails and the frequency of event A or practically a value close to the frequency is calculated. The probability value hence arrived is known as the statistical probability. In this case, the frequency of a certain event is 1 and the frequency of an impossible event is 0. Further, in a random event '*B*' which is the sum of events $A_1, A_2, \ldots., A_n$, the probability of B is given as $P(B) = P(A_1) + P(A_2) + \cdots + P(A_n)$. Also, for any random event A, $0 \leq P(A) \leq 1$.

Further, it is important to understand the distribution functions associated with the random variables. In order to specify a random variable, it is necessary to know the values or the range of values which it may assume. Hence it is important to know how the values are distributed. Suppose, Y is a random variable and x is an arbitrary real number, the probability that Y will take a value less than x is known as the distribution function of probabilities of the random variable Y.

$$F(x) = P\{Y < x\}$$

In another class of random variables, there is a nonnegative function $P(x)$ that satisfies the relation: For any x,

$$F(x) = \int_{-\infty}^{x} P(z)dz.$$

Such random variables are known as continuous and $P(x)$ is known as the probability density function. This density function has the properties:

$$P(x) \geq 0,$$

For any x_1 *and* $x_2, P\{x_1 \leq Y < x_2\} = \int_{x_1}^{x_2} P(x)dx$

$$\int P(x)dx = 1$$

In the case of a normal distribution, the density function is given as,

$$P(x) = Ce^{-\left(\frac{(x-\alpha)^2}{2\sigma^2}\right)}$$

where, C is a constant and is estimated using,

$$C\int e^{-\left(\frac{(x-\alpha)^2}{2\sigma^2}\right)}dx = 1$$

Let $\dfrac{x-\alpha}{\sigma} = z$, then:

$$C\sigma\int e^{-\left(\frac{z^2}{2}\right)}dz = 1$$

where $\int e^{-\left(\frac{z^2}{2}\right)}dz = \sqrt{2\pi}$, is the Poisson integral and hence:

$$C = \frac{1}{\sigma\sqrt{2\pi}}.$$

and hence, the normal distribution becomes,

$$P(x) = \frac{1}{\sigma\sqrt{2\pi}} e^{-\left(\frac{(x-\alpha)^2}{2\sigma^2}\right)}.$$

If $x = \alpha$, then $P(x)$ attains a maximum. The parameter σ has an effect on the shape of the curve and typical plots are shown in Figure 1.1 a–d.

1.2 ENTROPY

In order to do work, energy is consumed and this process generates a residual low quality energy which reduces the environmental quality. This irreversibility of the degradation of environment was discovered by Clausius and the residual energy is known as entropy, in the second law of thermodynamics. Several scientists have given different interpretations and definitions to entropy and are now applied in a variety of fields of science and engineering.

1.2.1 The Thermodynamic Entropy

In the field of statistical thermodynamics, the uncertainty of molecular states of a perfect gas is expressed in terms of entropy (Cropper, 1986; Naderi, 2010; Maroney, 2009). According to Boltzmann, the entropy of a perfect gas, changing states in an isothermal manner and at temperature T is expressed as:

$$S = -K\int_x \frac{(\psi - H)}{KT} \exp\{(\psi - H)/KT\}dx \tag{1}$$

where, ψ is the Gibb's energy and,

$$\psi = -KT \ln \exp\left\{\frac{-H}{KT}\right\},$$

where, H is the total energy of the system, and K is the Boltzmann's constant. For simplifying this problem, a probabilistic model is assumed in which entropy is a measure of the molecular distribution. Let $P(X)$ be the probability of a molecule being in state X, then

$$P(X) = \exp\{(\psi - H/kT\} \tag{2}$$

Substituting (2) in (1), we get,

$$S = -k\int_x P(X)\ln P(X)dx \tag{3}$$

This equation provides the definition of entropy as a measure of the uncertainty of the state of the system.

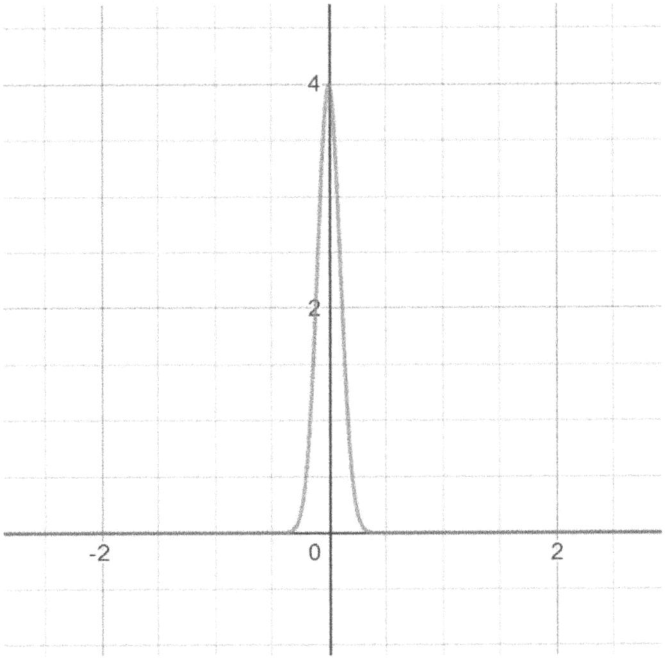

(a) normal distribution $\alpha = 0$, $\sigma = 0.1$

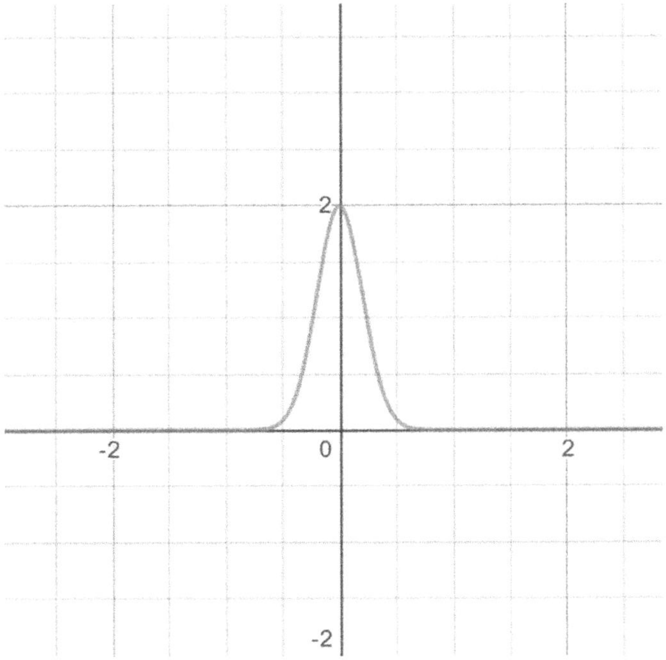

(b) normal distribution $\alpha = 0$, $\sigma = 0.2$

FIGURE 1.1 Normal distribution with different α and σ values

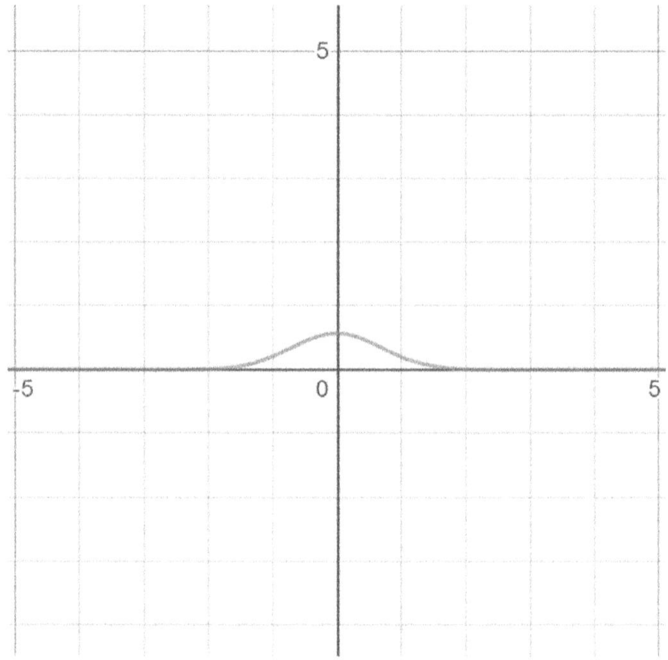

(c) normal distribution $\alpha = 0$, $\sigma = 0.7$

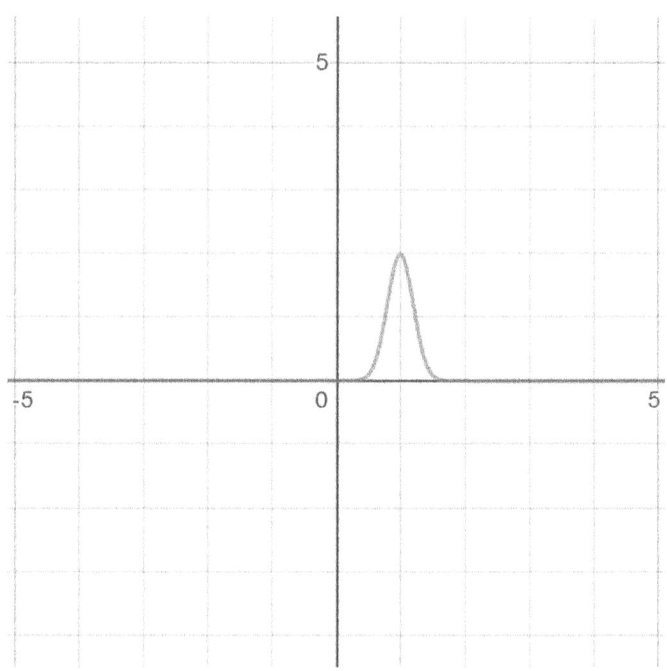

(d) normal distribution $\alpha = 1$, $\sigma = 0.2$

FIGURE 1.1 *(continued)*

1.2.2 Entropy in Information Theory

Entropy delivers highly insightful descriptions of the long-range behaviour of random processes (Cerf & Adami, 1997; Gray, 2011; Ambikapathy & Krishnamurthy, 2018). Using the principles of entropy provided by Boltzmann, the definition was extended to information theory by Shannon (Lesne, 2014). Shannon describes entropy as a measure of the uncertainty of the transmission of information.

$$H = -k \int_{\Omega} P(S) \ln P(S) dS$$

where, *P*(*S*) is a Gaussian density function over the space Ω of the transmitted information. Also, Shannon's definitions were further generalized to give rise to several definitions which enable the use of entropy in several areas of signal and image processing and analysis. Further, the entropy can be viewed as the degree of uncertainty or disorder or complexity associated with a system.

In the discrete sense, the Shannon's entropy can be approximated as,

$$H(X) = -C \sum_{i=1}^{n} P_i \log P_i$$

which enables the easy computation of the entropy of a variable or a set of values given by *X*. For example, consider a set of values assumed to be measured over a certain period, with the values given as *X* = [1, 1, 1, 2, 2, 2, 3, 3, 3, 3]. In order to compute the entropy, the frequency (*f*) or the number of times a certain value occurs is found out. In this case, the value 1 occurs 3 times, 2 occurs 3 times and 3 occurs 4 times. Hence the frequency of 1 is 3, the frequency of 2 is 3 and the frequency of 3 is 4.

Since there are total of 10 values, the probability of occurrence is given by,

$$P_i = f/N = f/10$$

Hence,

$$P_i(1) = 3/10 = 0.3,$$

$$P_i(2) = 3/10 = 0.3,$$

$$P_i(3) = 4/10 = 0.4.$$

Thus, the Shannon's entropy *H*(*X*) is computed as,

$$H(X) = -\left[0.3\log_2 0.3 + 0.3\log_2 0.3 + 0.4\log_2 0.4\right]$$

The above example provides a clear picture of how the entropy is calculated over a set of measured values.

Consider a thermodynamic state (A) which can be realized in many ways (w) at the microscopic level. It can be seen that the difference of Boltzmann entropies $S(A) - S_{\max}$ is proportional to $\log_2(P(A))$ Hence,

$$S_{\max} - S(A) = K.I(A)$$

where, $I(A)$ denotes the probabilistic information associated with set A. Therefore, it is inferred that the Boltzmann entropy is not exactly the same as Shannon entropy but however is closer to Shannon information.

For the analysis of signals and images, few more generalized representations are provided. The common measures being Tsallis and Renyi entropies.

1.2.3 Tsallis Entropy

The Tsallis entropy (Plastino & Plastino, 1999; dos Santos, 1997; Abe, 2002; Plastino & Plastino, 1994) in the continuous sense is given by:

$$H(q) = \frac{1 - \int ((f(x))^q \, dx}{q-1}$$

where, f is the probability density function.

The Tsallis entropy of a discrete system is given by:

$$H(q) = \frac{1 - \sum_{i=1}^{n} p_i^q}{q-1}$$

where, p is a probability distribution and q is a real number.

However, one can find that the Tsallis entropy converges to the Shannon's entropy when $q = 1$ (Maszczyk & Duch, 2008).

$$\lim_{q \to 1} H(q) = -\sum_{i=1}^{n} p_i \ln p_i$$

and

$$\lim_{q \to 1} H(q) = -\int f(x) \ln f(x) dx.$$

Tsallis entropy is hence a generalized representation of Shannon's entropy.

1.2.4 Renyi Entropy

The Renyi entropy (Lake, 2005; Bromiley et al.,2004; Golshani et al.,2009; Sahoo & Arora, 2004) of order α is defined as,

$$H(\alpha)=\frac{1}{1-\alpha}\ln\left(\sum_{i-1}^{n}p_i^{\alpha}\right),\quad \alpha\geq 0$$

and is viewed as a measure of information of order α associated with the probability distribution p_i. It can be seen that the Renyi entropy converges to Shannon's entropy when $\alpha=1$.

$$\lim_{\alpha\to 1}H(\alpha)=-\sum p_i \ln p_i$$

1.2.5 Dynamical Entropy

The dynamical entropy is equal to the average gain in one step of information about the initial state (Chakrabarti & Ghosh, 2013). Further the dynamical entropy of a process depends on the future. If $P=(p_i)_{i\in N}$ is a probability vector, the information function associated with it is $I_P : N\to[0.\infty]$ and is defined as (Downarowicz, 2011):

$$I_P(i)=-\log p_i$$

The entropy of P is given by,

$$\begin{aligned}H(P)&=\sum_{i=1}^{\infty}p_i I_P(i)\\&=-\sum_{i=1}^{\infty}p_i\log(p_i)\\&=\sum_{i=1}^{\infty}\eta(p_i)\end{aligned}$$

where, H is a concave function.

Further, if a probability vector $P=(p_i)$ satisfies $\sum_{i=1}^{\infty}ip_i<\infty$, then $H(P)<\infty$.

1.2.6 Spectral Entropy

As the Shannon entropy deals with the signals in time domain, likewise the spectral entropy is the entropy of signals in frequency domain. To calculate the spectral entropy of a signal, it is needed to utilize the power spectrum of a signal. It is important to remember that the Shannon entropy is calculated using the probability distribution. It should be noted that a signal with more frequency components has more entropy. To compute the spectral entropy, the following equations are utilized. The normalized power spectrum of a signal is given by (Bakiya, & Kamalanand, 2018; Semmlow & Griffel, 2014),

$$Q(f)=\frac{PS(f)}{\sum PS(f)}$$

where, $Q(f)$ is the normalized power spectrum and $PS(f)$ is the power spectrum.

Further using the normalized power spectrum, the spectral entropy (E_m) is given by:

$$E_m = \sum_f H(f)$$

where,

$$H(f) = \frac{Q(f)\log\left(\frac{1}{Q(f)}\right)}{\log(N)}$$

1.3 CHAOS AND ENTROPY

Chaos is the property of a deterministic system in which there is periodic long term behaviour. Such systems exhibit high sensitivity and changes in long term behaviours due to small changes in the initial conditions, as shown in Figure 1.2. Chaotic signals are abundant in the field of biology and most of the signals recorded from the human physiological system exhibit chaotic behaviour (Skinner, 1992; Weiss, 1994; Golberger, 1996 & Coffey, 1998).

1.3.1 Lyapunov Exponents

The Lyapunov exponents are utilized for the identification of chaos in a signal or system (Sano & Sawada 1985; Pikovsky & Politi 2016). A positive Lyapunov exponent indicates the presence of chaos. Consider two trajectories starting very close to each other, which will rapidly diverge away from each other to have very different futures. In such a case, the prediction over a long period of time is impossible. Consider $x(t)$ is a point at time t and consider a nearby point $x(t)+\delta(t)$, where δ is

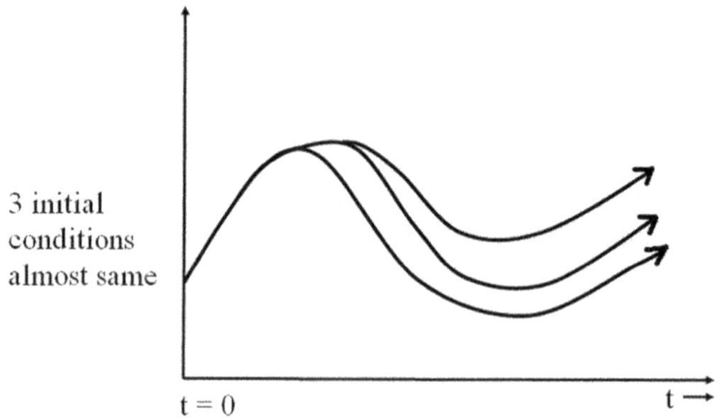

FIGURE 1.2 Changes in long term behaviour due to small changes in the initial conditions

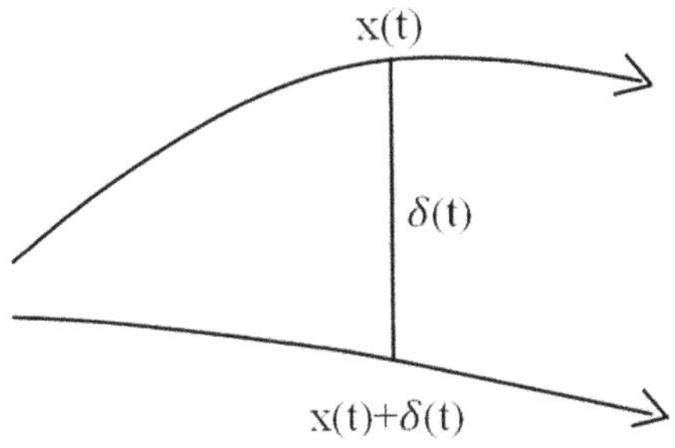

FIGURE 1.3 Two trajectories separated by a small value

a small separation of initial length $\|\delta_0\|$ equal to a very small value (say 10^{-10}) and $\|\delta(t)\| \sim \|\delta_0\| e^{\lambda t}$, as shown in Figure 1.3.

Plotting $\ln\|\delta\|$ as a function of time, the slope of the curve (λ) is known as the Lyapunov exponent, as shown in Figure 1.4. If the Lypunov exponent is negative, then the system exhibits random behaviour, if the value is positive, then the system exhibits chaotic behaviour (Shi, 2006). If the value is 0, a cyclic behaviour is implied.

Consider a dynamic model of a signal of the form,

$$x(k) = f(x(k-1)), \quad k = 1,2,3,...$$

Where, x is the signal amplitude at k^{th} instant and $f(.)$ is continuously differentiable, then the system linearized around the operational trajectory in the phase space can be given as:

$$\delta x(k) = J_{k-1} \delta x(k-1)$$

where,

$$J_{k-1} = \left. \frac{\partial f}{\partial x} \right|_{x_{k-1}} \in R^{mxm}, \quad k = 1,2,...$$

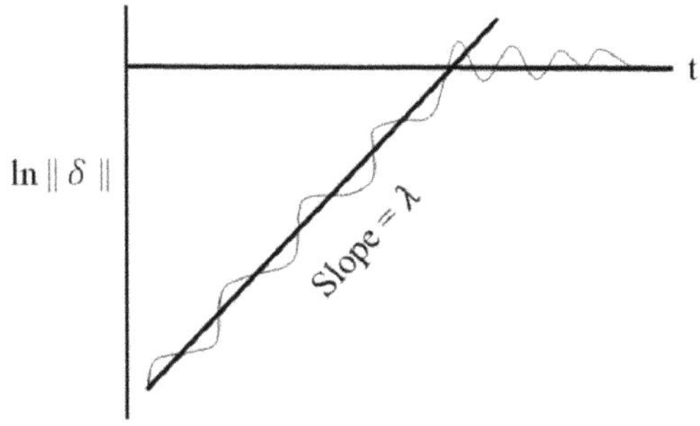

FIGURE 1.4 Estimation of the Lyapunov exponent

where, J_k is the Jacobean matrix at k. If $Y^k = J_{k-1}, J_{k-2}, \ldots J_0$, then a symmetric positive definite matrix can be defined as (Wu & Baleanu, 2015):

$$A = \lim_{k \to x} \left(\left(Y^k \right)^T Y^k \right)^{\frac{1}{2k}}$$

and the logarithms of the Eigen values of A are also known as the Lyapunov exponents.

Hence, the Lyapunov exponent actually quantifies the sensitivity to initial conditions in a dynamical system (Lai & Chen, 1998). Considering two trajectories with different initial conditions, close to each other, the trajectories diverge in the case of a chaotic attractor, at an exponential rate defined by the largest Lyapunov exponent. This can be generalized for a spectrum of Lyapunov exponents $\lambda_i, i = 1, 2, \ldots, n$, by considering several initial conditions in a small n-dimensional sphere. Let n be the number of state variables, and over a period of time, this sphere will evolve into an ellipsoid whose principal axes will change at different rates, described by the Lyapunov exponents. In this case, a single positive Lyapunov exponent confirms the presence of chaos in the system. From an information theoretic point of view, the information change in the system is given as a variation of the volume due to the changing principal axis. The sum of the positive Lyapunov exponents is equal to the Kolmogorov entropy which defines the mean rate of gain in information (Young, 1982).

$$\text{Kolmogorov entropy, } (K) = \sum_{\lambda_i > 0} \lambda_i$$

Hence, it is important to note that the well-established relationship exists between the Lyapunov exponent and the entropy of the system under investigation.

Another method of calculation of the Lyapunov exponents involves the reconstruction of the attractor dynamics from a signal or a given time series $x(t)$. The reconstructed trajectory (X), is expressed as a matrix where each row is a phase-space vector (Rosenstein et al., 1993).

$$X = \left[X_1, X_2, \ldots\ldots, X_M \right]^T$$

where, X_i is the state of the system at time i. For an N-point time series, $\{X_1, X_2, \ldots, X_N\}$, each X_i is given by,

$$X_i = \left[X_i,\ X_{i+J},\ \ldots,\ X_{i+(m-1)J} \right]$$

where, J is the lag or reconstruction delay, and m is the embedding dimension. Thus, X is an Mxm matrix and

$$M = N - (m-1)J$$

The embedding dimension is usually estimated in such a way that $m > 2n$. The lag or reconstruction delay, *J*, is equal to the lag where the autocorrelation function drops to 1- (1/e) of its initial value. The nearest neighbour $X_{\hat{j}}$ is found by searching for the point that minimizes the distance to the particular reference point, X_j. This is expressed as,

$$d_j(0) = \min X_j \left\| X_j - X_{\hat{j}} \right\|$$

where, $d_j(0)$ is the initial distance from the jth point to its nearest neighbour, and $\|.\|$ denotes the Euclidean norm. The largest Lyapunov exponent is then estimated as the mean rate of separation of the nearest neighbours. The Lyapunov exponents are expressed as:

$$\lambda_1(i) = \frac{1}{i.\Delta t} \cdot \frac{1}{(M-i)} \sum_{j=1}^{M-i} \ln \frac{d_j(i)}{d_j(0)}$$

where, *t* is the sampling period of the time series, and $d_j(i)$ is the distance between the jth pair of nearest neighbours after *i* discrete-time steps (Rosenstein et al., 1993).

1.3.2 Hurst Exponents

Further in the field of the study of chaos, another parameter known as the Hurst exponent can be defined. The Hurst exponent is a measure of the predictability of a time series or a signal. The Hurst exponent (*H*) in the range of 0.5 to 1, indicates correlated or persistent behaviour whereas *H* in the range of 0 to 0.5 denotes anti-persistent behaviour. A straight line with non-zero gradient will have $H = 1$ and a value of 0.5 will indicate an uncorrelated process or a white noise (Fernández-Martínez et al., 2014).

For estimation of the Hurst exponents, there are several procedures available. The most simple method being the detrended moving average in which a moving average $\tilde{y}_\omega(i)$ of a discrete signal $y(i)$, $i = 1, 2, ...N$,

where,

$$\tilde{y}_\omega(i) = \frac{1}{\omega} \sum_{k=0}^{\omega-1} y(i-k)$$

The trend of the signal is captured by the moving window $\omega \in [\omega_{\min}, \omega_{\max}]$. In the next step, the variance of $y(i)$ with respect to $\tilde{y}_\omega(i)$ is given as:

$$\sigma_i^2 = \frac{1}{\omega_{\max} - \omega} \sum_{i=\omega}^{\omega_{\max}} [y(i) - \tilde{y}_\omega(i)]^2$$

And since $\sigma \sim \omega^H$, *H* is calculated as a slope of the linear fit in the $\ln\sigma$, $\ln\omega$ plane.

In other method of estimation of the Hurst exponent known as the R/S method, a time series signal with N observations for specific intervals of time is divided to M sub-periods. The mean and standard deviation of each sub-period is given by:

$$\mu_m = \frac{1}{t}\sum_{k=1}^{n} N_{k,m}$$

$$S_m = \sqrt{\frac{1}{t}\sum_{k=1}^{n}(N_{k.m} - \mu_m)^2}$$

Further, the accumulated deviations are given as:

$$X_{k.m} = \sum_{k=1}^{n}(N_{k,m} - \mu_m)$$

and the amplitude of the mean deviations accumulated in each sequence I_m is given as:

$$R_m = \max(X_{k,m}) - \min(X_{k,m})$$

and finally we get:

$$R/S_t = \left[\left(\frac{1}{m}\right)\sum_{m=1}^{M}(R_m/S_m)\right]$$
$$= Ct^H$$

where, C is a constant, and

$$\log(R/S_t) = \log(C) + H\log(t).$$

Finally, the Hurst exponent (H) is estimated using a linear regression. Some of the available methods of estimation of Hurst exponents include the Residuals of regression method, Higuchi's method, Difference Variance method, Modified periodogram method, Aggregate variance method and Absolute moment method (Vialar, 2009; Zhou et al. 2007; Sun et al. 2008; Gospodinov & Gospodinova, 2005; Cervantes-De la Torre et al. 2013; Stroe-Kunold et al. 2009). However, it must be noted that there can be small variations in the Hurst exponent of a time series, computed using different methods as illustrated in an example in section 2.5 of Chapter 2.

1.3.3 Fractal Dimension

The fractal dimension of a signal or time series is a measure of the roughness or self-similarity of the series and is treated as an estimate of the local memory of the time series (Smith & Lange, 1998). The fractal dimension denoted by D has a value between $1 < D \leq 2$ for univariate series. The relationship between fractal dimension and the Hurst exponent is well established and is given by (Chen et al., 2011)

$$D + H = 2$$

If the fractal dimension value is less than 1.5, then the series is less rough and a high fractal dimension with $D > 1.5$ represents a rough series.

Another method of estimating fractal dimension of a signal or time series is the Higuchi's algorithm (Gómez et al., 2009). Consider a set of measurements recorded at regular time intervals:

$$X(1), X(2), ..., X(N)$$

From the measured series, a new series $X_k{}^m$ is constructed as follows:

$$X_k^m;\ X(m), X(m+1), X(m+2), ..., X\left(m + \left[\frac{N-m}{K}\right]k\right)$$

where, m = 1, 2, …, k and m indicate the initial time and k denotes the interval time. Then the length of the curve associated to each of the time series $X_k{}^m$ is represented by:

$$L_m(k) = \frac{1}{k} \sum_{i=1}^{\left[\frac{n-m}{K}\right]} (X(m+ik) - X(M+(i-1)k) \left(\frac{N-1}{\left[\frac{N-m}{K}\right]k} \right)$$

and $\frac{N-1}{\left[\frac{N-m}{K}\right]k}$ is a normalization factor.

Then the average value $\langle L(k) \rangle$ of the associated lengths is calculated and this average follows a power law:

$$\langle L(k) \rangle \alpha\, k^{-D}$$

where, D is the fractal dimension.

1.3.4 Spectral Exponents

Any given signal can be represented as the superposition of periodic signals and a time series or signal $X(t)$ in an interval T with mean given by (Colombo et al., 2019):

$$\bar{X}(t) = \frac{1}{T} \int_0^1 X(t)dt$$

and variance σ^2 is given by:

$$\sigma^2(X(t)) = \frac{1}{T}\int_0^1 \left[X(t) - \bar{X}(t)\right]^2 dt.$$

This series can be represented in the frequency domain by:

$$A(f,t)) = \int_{-\infty}^{\infty} X(t)e^{2\pi ift}dt$$

which is the Fourier transform of $X(t)$ and the inverse Fourier transform is given as:

$$X(t) = \int_{-\infty}^{\infty} A(f,t)e^{-2\pi ift}df.$$

Further, the spectral power density is given as:

$$S(f) = \lim_{T\to\infty}\frac{1}{T}|A(f,t)|^2.$$

In a fractal time series, the power law relation is satisfied:

$$S(f)\alpha f^{-\beta}$$

where, β is known as the spectral exponent and can be used to characterize the dynamic behaviour of the time series.

$\beta = 0$ occurs in the case of white noise and $\beta = 1$ occurs in moderately correlated system and $\beta = 2$ is observed in Brownian noise.

It is interesting to note that the spectral exponent β is related to the fractal dimension D by:

$$\beta = 5 - 2D$$

Further, if $1 \le \beta \le 3$, then $D = \frac{5-\beta}{2}$ and also if $\beta \to 0$ then $D \to 2$ and if $\beta \to 3$ then $D \to 1$.

It has to be noted that there is a strong relation between the Shannon entropy and the fractal dimension (Ampilova & Soloviev, 2018)

1.4 ENTROPY OF BIOLOGICAL SYSTEMS

The process of life happens due to multiple chemical reactions taking place in every organism. In this process, the organisms tend to store or spend energy and there is a continuous transfer of heat from the organism to the surroundings due to the metabolic activities. Since the chemical reactions in the living organisms are exothermic, there is a continuous evolution of heat in living processes (Aoki, 2001). However, in some undesired state of biological systems such as cancer, more heat is generated compared to the normal. Since entropy is one of the most important quantities in nature, the entropy of biological systems can be correlated with the aging process and life itself. Some basic properties of entropy are well correlated with biological processes (Mitrokhin,2014; Baez & Pollard, 2016; Daniel, 2009):

- Entropy is a measure of the disorder
- Entropy increases with increase in the size of the system
- Excess entropy production implies the speed of progression towards equilibrium.

1.5 MUTUAL INFORMATION

The mutual information is a quantitate measure of the shared information between two signals. Since there are several biosignals in the human body and all signals are well correlated with each other, it is always important to quantify the mutual information between such signals. In order to estimate the mutual information of two correlated events, it is necessary to find their individual probability distribution and also their joint probability distribution. Consider a signal $x[n]$ with m potential states. For this signal, the probability of finding a particular value at any sample n is equal to $p(x_m)$ which is the probability distribution function for any of the m potential states. Also considering another signal $y(n)$ with k potential states, and the probability distribution function is $p(y_k)$ or $p(y)$ and the joint distribution function between the signals is $p(x, y)$, the information present in the joint event is given by:

$$H_{xy} = -\sum_{mk} p(x, y) \log_2 p(x, y)$$

And the mutual information of these signals is given by:

$$\begin{aligned} MI_{xy} &= H_x + H_y - H_{xy} \\ &= \sum_{mk} p(x, y) \log_2 \frac{p(x, y)}{p(x)p(y)} \end{aligned}$$

where, $p(x.y)$ is the probability of the events in these signals happening simultaneously (Semmlow & Griffel, 2014).

REFERENCES

Abe, S.(2002). Stability of Tsallis entropy and instabilities of Rényi and normalized Tsallis entropies: a basis for q-exponential distributions. *Physical Review E*, 6(4), 046134.

Ambikapathy, B., & Krishnamurthy, K. (2018). Analysis of electromyograms recorded using invasive and noninvasive electrodes: a study based on entropy and lyapunov exponents estimated using artificial neural networks. *Journal of Ambient Intelligence and Humanized Computing*, 1–9.

Ampilova, N., & Soloviev, I.(2018). Entropies in investigation of dynamical systems and their application to digital image analysis. *Journal of Measurements in Engineering*, 6(2), 107–118.

Aoki, I. (2001). Entropy and exergy principles in living systems. In *Thermodynamics and Ecological Modelling* (pp. 167–190). Lewis Publishers.

Baez, J. C., & Pollard, B. S. (2016). Relative entropy in biological systems. *Entropy*, 18(*2*), 46.

Bakiya, A., & Kamalanand, K. (2018). Information analysis on electromyograms acquired using monopolar needle, concentric needle and surface electrodes. In *2018 International Conference on Recent Trends in Electrical, Control and Communication (RTECC)* (pp. 240–244). IEEE.

Bromiley, P. A., Thacker, N. A., & Bouhova-Thacker, E. (2004). Shannon entropy, Renyi entropy, and information. *Statistics and Inf. Series (2004-004).*

Brooks, D. R., Collier, J., Maurer, B. A., Smith, J. D., & Wiley, E. O. (1989). Entropy and information in evolving biological systems. *Biology and Philosophy*, 4(*4*), 407–432.

Cerf, N. J., & Adami, C. (1997). Negative entropy and information in quantum mechanics. *Physical Review Letters*, 79(*26*), 5194.

Cervantes-De la Torre, F., González-Trejo, J. I., Real-Ramirez, C. A., & Hoyos-Reyes, L. F. (2013). Fractal dimension algorithms and their application to time series associated with natural phenomena. *Journal of Physics: Conference Series*, 475(1), 012002.

Chakrabarti, C. G., & Ghosh, K. (2013). Dynamical entropy via entropy of non-random matrices: application to stability and complexity in modelling ecosystems. *Mathematical Biosciences*, 245(*2*), 278–281.

Chen, C. C., Lee, Y. T., Hasumi, T., & Hsu, H. L. (2011). Transition on the relationship between fractal dimension and Hurst exponent in the long-range connective sandpile models. *Physics Letters A*, 375(*3*), 324–328.

Coffey, D. S. (1998). Self-organization, complexity and chaos: the new biology for medicine. *Nature Medicine*, 4(*8*), 882–885.

Colombo, M. A., Napolitani, M., Boly, M., Gosseries, O., Casarotto, S., Rosanova, M., & Massimini, M. (2019). The spectral exponent of the resting EEG indexes the presence of consciousness during unresponsiveness induced by propofol, xenon, and ketamine. *Neuroimage*, *189*, 631–644.

Cropper, W. H. (1986). Rudolf clausius and the road to entropy. *American Journal of Physics*, 54(*12*), 1068–1074.

Daniel, H. (2009). *Entropy Theory of Aging Systems: Humans, Corporations and the Universe*. World Scientific.

dos Santos, R. J. (1997). Generalization of Shannon's theorem for Tsallis entropy. *Journal of Mathematical Physics*, 38(*8*), 4104–4107.

Downarowicz, T. (2011). *Entropy in Dynamical Systems (New Mathematical Monographs).* Cambridge University Press.

Fernández-Martínez, M., Sánchez-Granero, M. A., Segovia, J. T., & Román-Sánchez, I. M. (2014). An accurate algorithm to calculate the hurst exponent of self-similar processes. *Physics Letters A*, 378(*32-33*), 2355–2362.

Frank, S. A., & Smith, D. E. (2010). Measurement invariance, entropy, and probability. *Entropy*, 12(*3*), 289–303.

Gladyshev, G. P. (1999). On thermodynamics, entropy and evolution of biological systems: what is life from a physical chemist's viewpoint. *Entropy*, 1(*2*), 9–20.

Golberger, A. L. (1996). Non-linear dynamics for clinicians: chaos theory, fractals, and complexity at the bedside. *The Lancet*, 347(*9011*), 1312–1314.

Golshani, L., Pasha, E., & Yari, G.(2009). Some properties of Rényi entropy and Rényi entropy rate. *Information Sciences*, 179(*14*), 2426–2433.

Gómez, C., Mediavilla, Á, Hornero, R., Abásolo, D., & Fernández, A. (2009). Use of the Higuchi's fractal dimension for the analysis of MEG recordings from Alzheimer's disease patients. *Medical Engineering & Physics*, 31(*3*), 306–313.
Gospodinov, M., & Gospodinova, E. (2005). The graphical methods for estimating hurst parameter of self-similar network traffic. In *Proceedings of the 2005 International Conference on Computer Systems and Technologies* (pp. 1–6). ACM.
Gray, R. M. (2011). *Entropy and Information Theory*. Springer Science & Business Media.
Kamalanand, K., & Jawahar, P. (2018). *Mathematical Modelling of Systems and Analysis*. PHI Learning Pvt. Ltd.
Kvålseth, T. O.(2016). On the measurement of randomness (uncertainty): a more informative entropy. *Entropy*, 18(*5*), 159.
Lai, D., & Chen, G.(1998). Statistical analysis of lyapunov exponents from time series: ajacobian approach. *Mathematical and Computer Modelling*, 27(*7*), 1–9.
Lake, D. E. (2005). Renyi entropy measures of heart rate gaussianity. *IEEE Transactions on Biomedical Engineering*, 53(*1*), 21–27.
Lesne, A. (2014). Shannon entropy: a rigorous notion at the crossroads between probability, information theory, dynamical systems and statistical physics. *Mathematical Structures in Computer Science*, *24*(3).
Maassen, H., & Uffink, J. B. (1988). Generalized entropic uncertainty relations. *Physical Review Letters*, 60(*12*), 1103.
Maroney, O. (2009). Information processing and thermodynamic entropy.
Martyushev, L. M., & Seleznev, V. D. (2006). Maximum entropy production principle in physics, chemistry and biology. *Physics Reports*, 426(*1*), 1–45.
Maszczyk, T., & Duch, W. (2008, June). Comparison of Shannon, Renyi and Tsallis entropy used in decision trees. In *International Conference on Artificial Intelligence and Soft Computing* (pp. 643–651). Springer, Berlin, Heidelberg.
Mitrokhin, Y. (2014). Two faces of entropy and information in biological systems. *Journal of Theoretical Biology*, *359*, 192–198.
Naderi, M., Amiri, M., & Khonsari, M. M. (2010). On the thermodynamic entropy of fatigue fracture. *Proceedings of the Royal Society A: Mathematical, Physical and Engineering Sciences*, 466(*2114*), 423–438.
Pikovsky, A., & Politi, A. (2016). *Lyapunov Exponents: A Tool to Explore Complex Dynamics*. Cambridge University Press.
Plastino, A. R. P. A., & Plastino, A. R. (1999). Tsallis entropy and Jaynes' information theory formalism. *Brazilian Journal of Physics*, 29(*1*), 50–60.
Plastino, A. R., & Plastino, A. (1994). Dynamical aspects of Tsallis' entropy. *Physica A: Statistical Mechanics and its Applications*, 202(*3-4*), 438–448.
Rosenstein, M. T., Collins, J. J., & De Luca, C. J. (1993). A practical method for calculating largest lyapunov exponents from small data sets. *Physica D: Nonlinear Phenomena*, 65(*1-2*), 117–134.
Sahoo, P. K., & Arora, G. (2004). A thresholding method based on two-dimensional Renyi's entropy. *Pattern Recognition*, 37(*6*), 1149–1161.
Sano, M., & Sawada, Y. (1985). Measurement of the lyapunov spectrum from a chaotic time series. *Physical Review Letters*, 55(*10*), 1082.
Semmlow, J. L., & Griffel, B. (2014). *Biosignal and Medical Image Processing*. CRC press.
Shi, W. (2006). Lyapunov exponent analysis to chaotic phenomena of marine power system. *IFAC Proceedings Volumes*, 39(*13*), 1497–1502.
Skinner, J. E., Molnar, M., Vybiral, T., & Mitra, M. (1992). Application of chaos theory to biology and medicine. *Integrative Physiological and Behavioral Science*, 27(*1*), 39–53.
Smith, T. G., & Lange, G. D. (1998). Biological cellular morphometry-fractal dimensions, lacunarity and multifractals. In *Fractals in biology and medicine* (pp. 30–49). Birkhäuser.

Stroe-Kunold, E., Stadnytska, T., Werner, J., & Braun, S. (2009). Estimating long-range dependence in time series: an evaluation of estimators implemented in R. *Behavior Research Methods*, 41(*3*), 909–923.

Sun, W., Rachev, S. Z., & Fabozzi, F. (2008). Long-range dependence, fractal processes, and intra-daily data. In *Handbook on Information Technology in Finance* (pp. 543). Springer, Berlin, Heidelberg.

Vialar, T. (2009). Complex and chaotic nonlinear dynamics. *Advances in Economics and Finance, Mathematics and Statistics, Springer.*

Wang, N., Li, Y., & Zhang, H. (2010). Hurst exponent estimation based on moving average method. In *Advances in Wireless Networks and Information Systems* (pp. 137). Springer, Berlin, Heidelberg.

Weiss, J. N., Garfinkel, A., Spano, M. L., & Ditto, W. L. (1994). Chaos and chaos control in biology. *The Journal of Clinical Investigation*, 93(*4*), 1355–1360.

Wilson, J. A. (1968). Increasing entropy of biological systems. *Nature*, 219(*5153*), 534–535.

Wu, G. C., & Baleanu, D. (2015). Jacobian matrix algorithm for lyapunov exponents of the discrete fractional maps. *Communications in Nonlinear Science and Numerical Simulation*, 22(*1-3*), 95–100.

Young, L. S. (1982). Dimension, entropy and lyapunov exponents. *Ergodic Theory and Dynamical Systems*, 2(*1*), 109–124.

Zhou, P., Li, F., Liu, W. Y., & Yang, M. (2007). Fractal analysis in normal EEG and epileptic EEG of rats. In *World Congress on Medical Physics and Biomedical Engineering 2006* (pp. 1266–1269). Springer, Berlin, Heidelberg.

2 Biosignals

Due to the recent advancement of semiconductor technology in the field of amplifiers and filters, several electrophysiological signals such as electrocardiograms (ECG), electro encephalograms (EEG), electroretinograms (ERG), electrooculograms (EOG), electromayograms (EMG) etc., are efficiently utilized for the effective diagnosis of the disorders associated with the physiological system (Naït-Ali 2009; Tranquillo, 2013).

2.1 CLASSIFICATION AND CHARACTERISTICS OF BIOSIGNALS

The biosignals can be viewed as a manifestation of the living process and they reflect the nature and activity of the physiological system (Escabí, 2012; Tranquillo, 2013). Further these signals can also reflect upon the state of the system including the pathologies associated with it (Liang, 2012; Gratton, 2007; Semmlow, 2017). Also, apart from electrical signals from the body, there are also other types of signals and can be listed and classified as follows:

- Bio electric signals (signals generated by nerve cells/action potentials)
- Bio acoustic signals (example: flow of blood, flow of air)
- Bio mechanical signals (motion/displacement/chest wall/respiratory activity)
- Bio magnetic signals (generated by the magnetic field of heart and brain)
- Bio chemical signals (0_2, Ph values)
- Bio optical signals (generated by transmission and reflection of light)

These signals represent the normal wellbeing of the system under investigation. However, any change in the characteristics of these signals represents altered performance or abnormal states of the system (Tranquillo, 2013). Based on the complexity of the bio signals, they can be classified into

- Less complex bio signal
- Moderate complex bio signal
- More complex bio signal

Further, based on a signal processing point of view, the bio signals are classified into three different types namely (Javadpour & Mohammadi, 2015; Harris, 1987; Toker, 2020):

1. The deterministic signals: These signals can be represented as a function and the future values of these signals can be predicted from their post values.

2. The stochastic signals: These signals are random in nature and it is not possible to predict the future values from the past values.
3. Chaotic signals: Theses signals exhibit complex properties such as chaos.

Further, fractal signals exhibit scale invariance in which a similar pattern repeats itself invariant to the scale in which it is studied.

2.2 MEASUREMENT OF BIOSIGNALS

The acquisition and analysis of biosignals and diagnosis of a particular disease, involves several stages as shown in Figure 2.1. The first stage involves the acquisition of the signal from the region of interest of the body. The region of interest can be a particular muscle or tissue or even a single cell (Escabí, 2005; Boashash, 2015).

This acquisition is made using the placement of a suitable physiological transducer (example: electrodes or microphones) on the location of interest. Further, the output of physiological transducer is amplified and filtered using suitable electronic circuits (Levkov, 1988; Lotte, 2007). For example, circuits are shown in Figure 2.2 and 2.3.

The next part involves in the conversion of the analogue signals into digital signals for storage and processing in a computer. Further, the signals are again processed using softwares for removal of artifacts and for the detection of events in the signals. Finally, the useful features are extracted from the signals for the development of automated diagnostic systems (Supratak et al., 2016). These features can be viewed as biomarkers which enable the classifications of the signals into normal and abnormal signals. The features can be as simple as the statistical descriptors such as the mean, median, variance, standard deviation, skewness and kurtosis (Tamil et al., 2008; Ahsan et al., 2009). Also, the features can be obtained using the processing of such signals using various algorithms. For example, the coefficients of the wavelet decomposition of the signals have been used as effective features for the classification of normal and abnormal biosignals (Dickhaus & Heinrich, 1996).

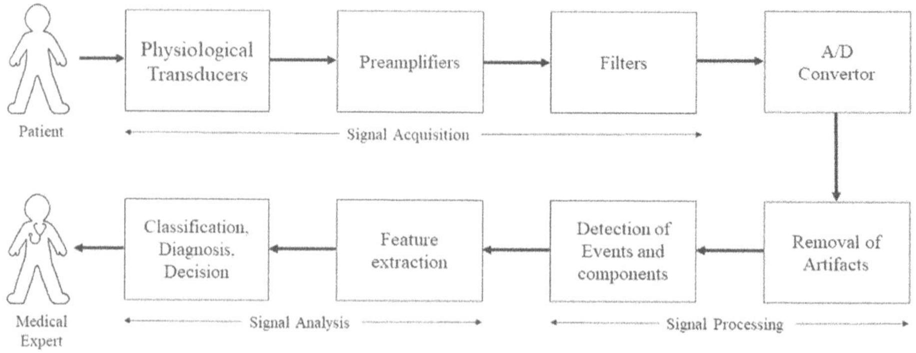

FIGURE 2.1 Recording and analysis of biosignals

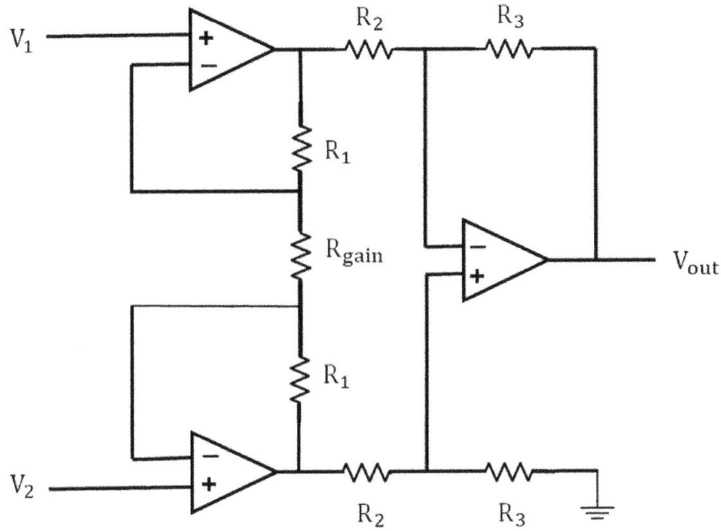

FIGURE 2.2 The circuit based on operational amplifiers for amplification of biosignals

However, when discussing about bio signals, it is important to mention the problems associated with recording these signals due to the following factors (Van Bemmel et al., 1997; Singh et al., 2012):

1. The effect of instrumentation and the procedure of recording on the physiological system. For example, the placement of surface electrodes on the skin for recording electrophysiological signals leads to the change in the overall impedance associated with the system.
2. Access of the variable to the measurement system.
3. Variability of signal source.
4. Artefacts due to breathing, body vibrations, motion, cross talk, ambient environment.
5. Energy limitations.
6. Patient safety (factors include shock and radiation hazards).

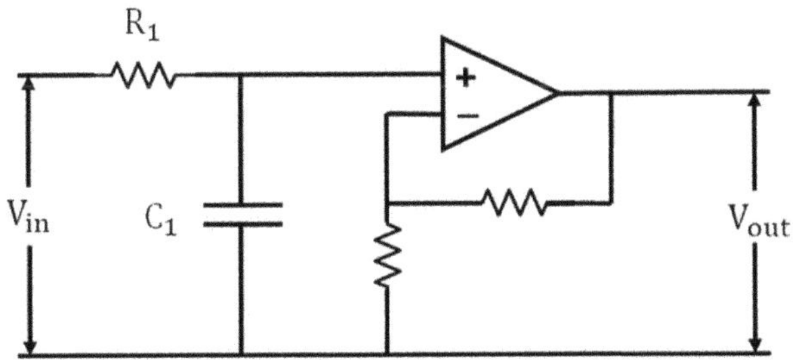

FIGURE 2.3 A low pass filter circuit for filtering biosignals

2.3 ENTROPY OF ELECTROPHYSIOLOGICAL SIGNALS

The entropy of biosignals offers a distinct demarcation between normal and abnormal states of the physiological system (Zhang, 2017; Pham, 2017; Castiglioni et al., 2013). At any given instant, a biosignal carries vital information about the health of the physiological system. This information can change over a period of time due to changes in the activity, aging and diseases/disorders of the physiological system. Hence, it is important to analyse the information or entropy associated with biosignals since it is the disorder associated with that system.

In dynamical systems, the entropy is the rate at which the signal loses or gains information. However, in the field of information theory, the analysis of entropy relates to the measurement of information content of the signal (Gray, 2011; Cerf & Adami, 1997). Signals which are cyclic or have a certain regularity associated with them have no large quantity of entropy. To illustrate this scenario, consider a sinusoidal wave of a particular amplitude and frequency. In such a signal, there is no associated information. This is the reason for high entropies in nonlinear systems when compared to linear systems. Due to the higher entropy in nonlinear systems such as the physiological system, these systems generate complex patterns like fractals and chaos (Carlen et al., 2008; Xue et al., 2011). The quantification of information become possible since the information content in signal is inversely proportional to measure the information content by measuring the uncertainty or complexity of a signal (Semmlow & Griffel, 2014).

Recently, researchers have utilized various entropic measures for analysis of the biosignal characteristics with respect to various abnormalities and also to analyse the characteristics of the measurement equipment (Jovic & Bogunovic, 2007; Chen et al., 2007; Srinivasan et al., 2007; Azami et al., 2017). In the areas of feature extraction, the entropic measures find an application and these measures have already been proved to be excellent features for the analysis of bio signals and also for the development of computer aided diagnostic systems for the automated diagnosis of several diseases.

2.3.1 The Entropy of Electromyograms

The muscoskeletal system in the human body is highly important as it facilitates the movement and maintains posture and balance. This system is controlled by the nervous system. The disorders associated with the muscular system can be due to a variety of conditions such as the myopathy (problems associated with the muscles) and neuropathy (problems associated with nerves) (Kugelberg, 1947; Cacioppo & Petty, 1981; Ahmad & Chappellm 2008; Ambikapathy & Krishnamurthy, 2018). Electromyography records the electrical signals generated by the nerves and the muscles (Bakiya et al., 2018; Ambikapathy et al., 2018). Since these signals are well correlated with the normal and abnormal states of the muscles, these EMG signals are utilized by the physicians to diagnose a variety of neuromuscular disorders (Bakiya, & Kamalanand, 2018). As an illustrative example, the entropic analysis on typical electromyogram (EMG) signals recorded from a normal subject and patients with myopathy and neuropathy and collected from the Physiobank opensource database of clinical signals, is presented. Figure 2.4 presents the normal, myopathy and neuropathy EMG signals.

The variation of the Renyi entropy of normal, myopathy and neuropathy EMG signals, is shown in Figure 2.5, as a function of the order of entropy (α) in the range of 0.1 to 0.9. It is observed that the Renyi entropy increases exponentially with increase in α in the range of 0.1 to 0.9. Significant variations in the magnitude of the

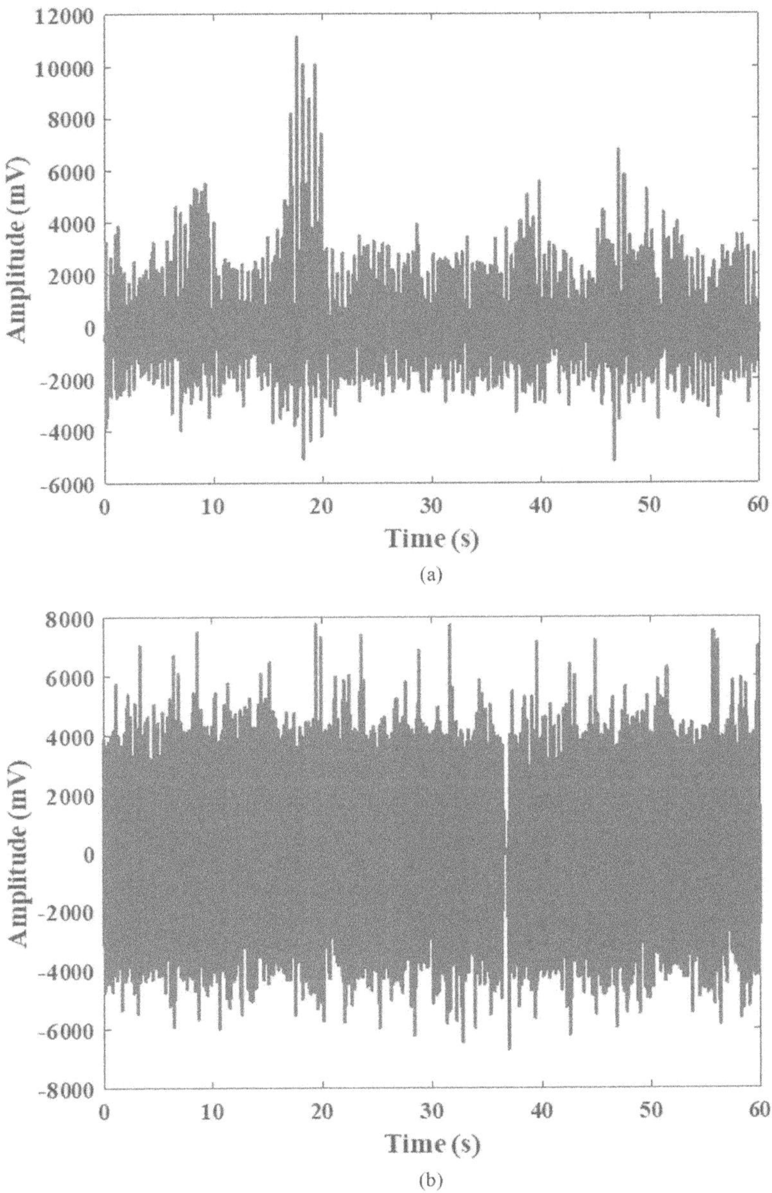

FIGURE 2.4 Typical (a) normal, (b) myopathy and (c) neuropathy electromyogram signals

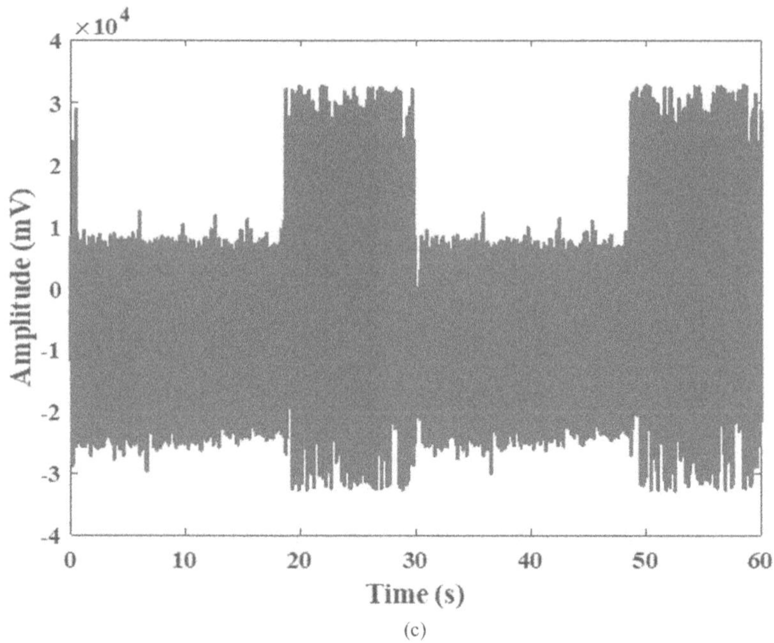

FIGURE 2.4 (*continued*)

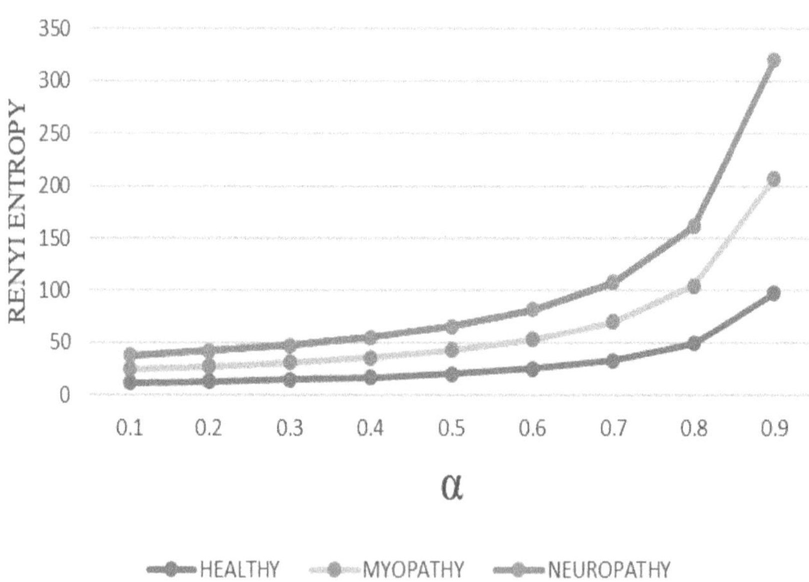

FIGURE 2.5 The variation of Renyi entropy of normal, myopathy and neuropathy EMG signals, shown as a function of α in the range of 0.1 to 0.9

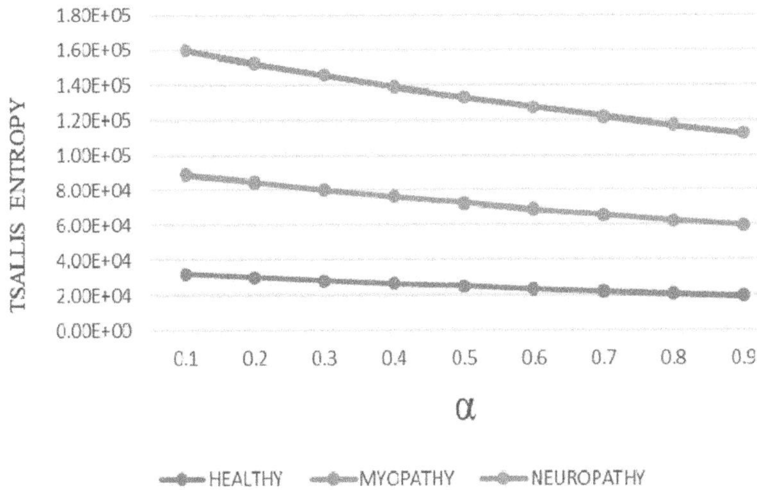

FIGURE 2.6 The variation of Tsallis entropy of normal, myopathy and neuropathy EMG signals, shown as a function of α in the range of 0.1 to 0.9

Renyi entropy are observed between the normal, myopathy and neuropathy EMG signals. The Renyi entropy of the abnormal EMG signals is found to be higher than the normal signals. Figure 2.6 shows the variation in the Tsallis entropy of normal, myopathy and neuropathy EMG signals, as a function of the order of entropy α in the range of 0.1 to 0.9. It can be seen that the Tsallis entropy values reduces linearly with increase in α. Similar to the Renyi entropy values, the Tsallis entropy values were found to be higher in the case of myopathy and neuropathy EMG signals when compared to the normal EMG signals. In the case of both Renyi entropy and Tsallis entropy, a significant variation can be observed between normal, myopathy and neuropathy EMG signals. These features have the potential to offer a distinct demarcation between the normal and abnormal classes hence can be utilized as a tool for diagnosis of muscle disorders using EMG signals.

Figure 2.7 shows the variation of the computed Tsallis entropy for the normal, myopathy and neuropathy EMG signal, for various values of α in the range of 0 to 9 in steps of 1. It can be observed that even though there are no measurable changes in the Tsallis entropy of normal and myopathy EMG signals, there is a significant difference between the Tsallis entropy of neuropathy EMG signals compared to the other two cases. The Tsallis entropy of normal and myopathic EMG signals decreases when α increases from 8 to 9. However, the Tsallis entropy increases in the case of neuropathy EMG signal, when α changes from 8 to 9.

2.3.2 Entropy of Gait Signals

Also, another illustrative example on the typical variations of Tsallis entropy of human gait signals recorded from patients with disorders namely Amyotrophic lateral sclerosis (ALS), Parkinson's Disease (PD) and Huntington's Disease (HD),

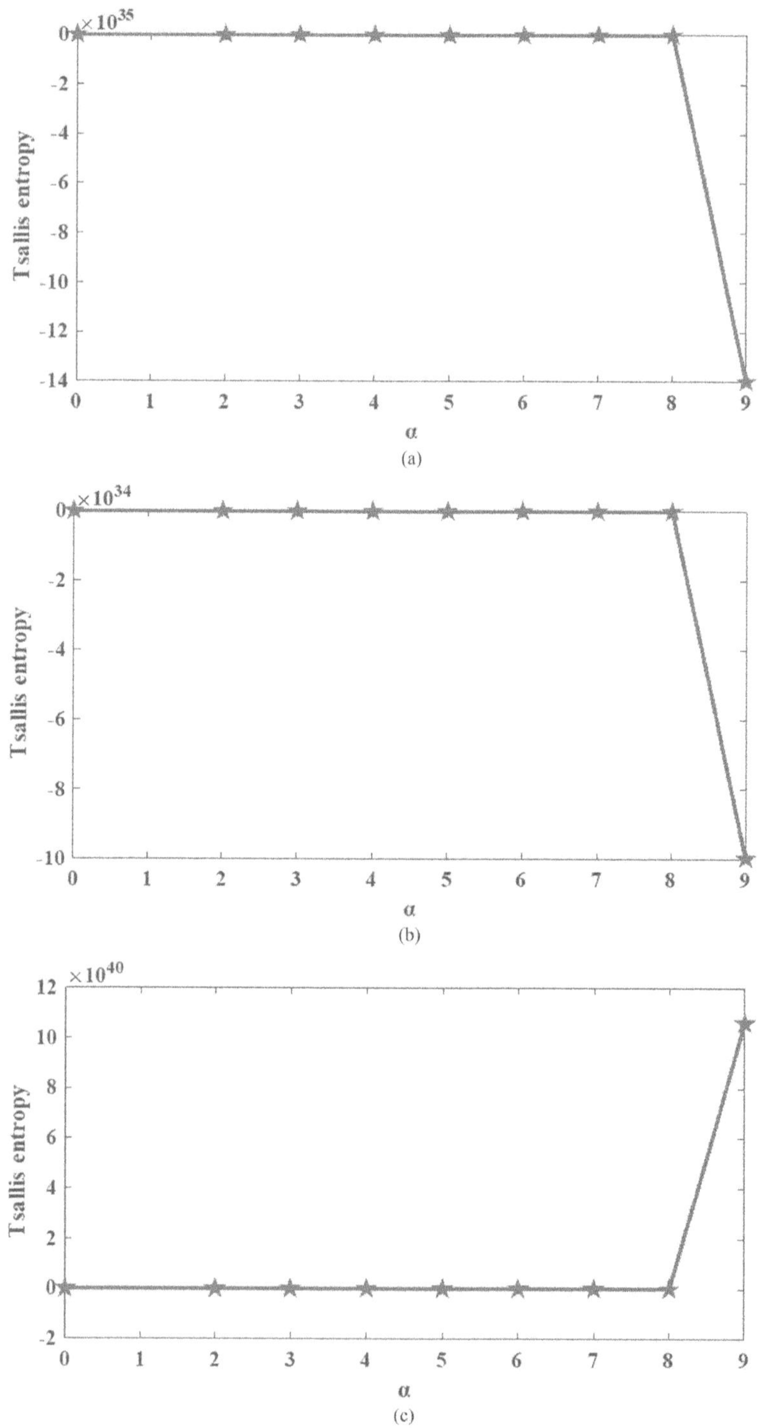

FIGURE 2.7 The variation of Tsallis entropy shown as a function of the order of entropy (α) for (a) normal, (b) myopathy and (c) neuropathy EMG signals

when compared to normal gait is presented (Brooks et al., 1988; Gil et al., 2010; Ren et al., 2015). The pattern of human locomotion is normally measured using gait signals. Human locomotion is the mechanism which is possible due to the inter connected activity of the bones, muscles in coordination with the nervous system (Dietz et al., 1979; Taga, 1995; Medved, 2000). The gait measurement system consists of instrumentation involving force sensors placed under the foot for measuring the body movements and mechanics. Commonly gait signals are utilized for

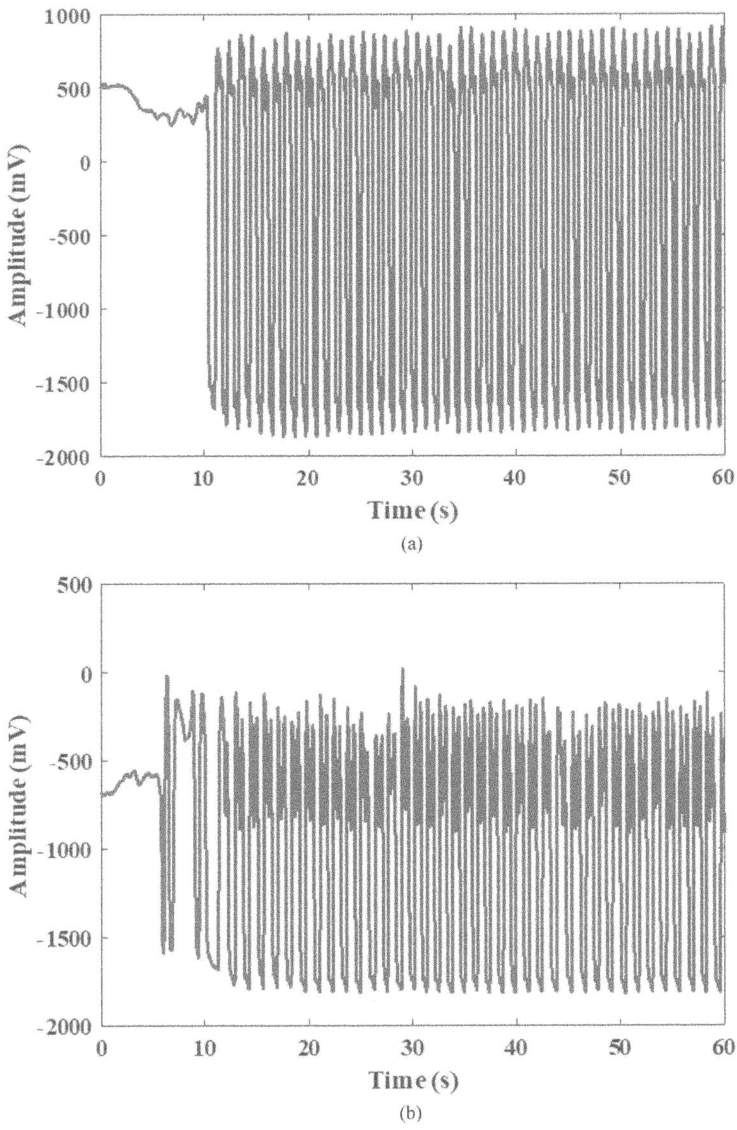

FIGURE 2.8 The typical left foot gait signals recorded from (a) normal subject, (b) patient with amyotrophic lateral sclerosis (ALS), (c) Parkinson's disease and (d) Huntington's disease

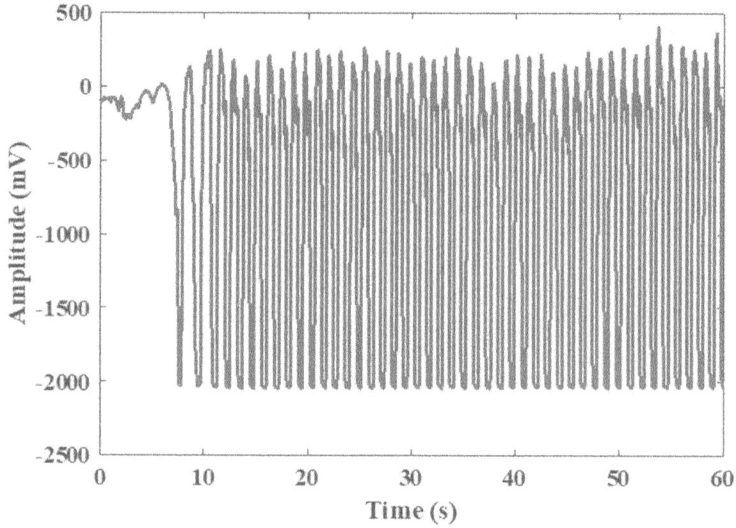

(c)

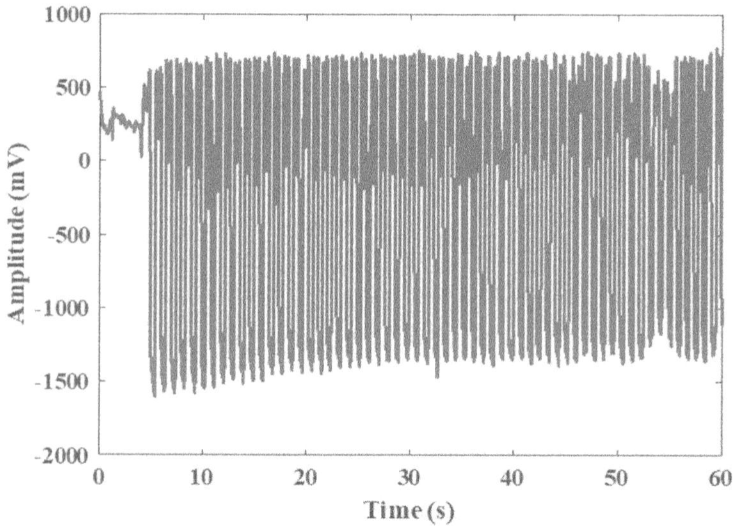

(d)

FIGURE 2.8 (*continued*)

analysing the physiological and pathological conditions of individuals (Shiavi et al., 1998; Sejdić et al., 2013). These associated problems affect their ability to walk and hence gait signals can be utilized to diagnose a variety of neurological, skeletal as well as muscular disorders. Apart from the pathological conditions, certain other features such as the terrain on which the individual is walking, footwear, sex, weight, height and age also induce variations in the gait pattern.

The gait signals recorded from the left foot, collected from the opensource database (PhysioBank) were analysed and Figure 2.8 shows the typical gait signal

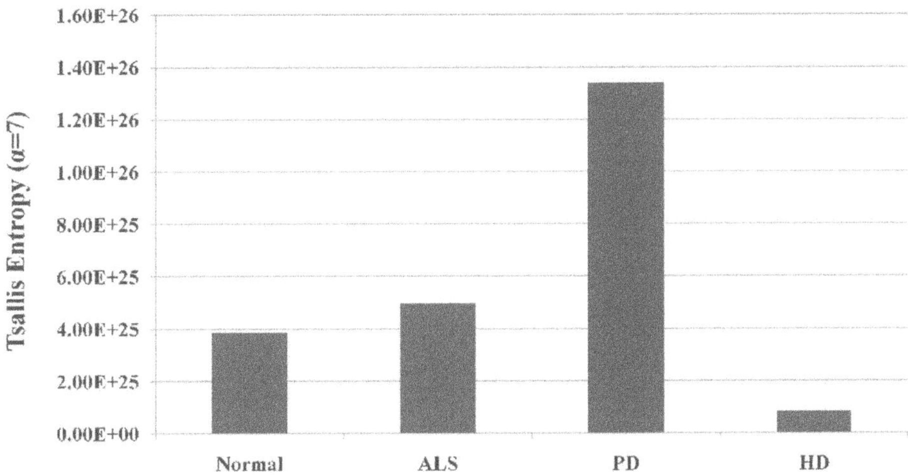

FIGURE 2.9 The variation of Tsallis entropy ($\alpha = 7$) of normal, ALS, PD and HD left foot gait signals

recorded from the left foot of a normal subject, patients with Amyotrophic lateral sclerosis (ALS), Parkinson's disease and Huntington's disease. Notable variations in the recorded signals can be observed between the considered disorders compared with the normal gait. The variation of the Tsallis entropy of order 7 for of normal, ALS, PD and HD left foot gait signals are presented in Figure 2.9. It is seen that there are significant differences in the magnitude of Tsallis entropy of order 7.

2.4 HJORTH INFORMATION

The Hjorth information included three different parameters which can be utilized for efficient characterization of bio signals. Activity, mobility and complexity of biosignals are the three parameters which provide information about the frequency as well as temporal characteristics of bio signals These parameters have been well utilized to extract useful information for the analysis and characterization of bio signals (Alagumariappan et al., 2020; Oh et al., 2014; Hamida et al., 2015; Damaševičius et al., 2018).

2.4.1 Hjorth Activity

The Hjorth activity describes the variance of bio signal. In a broad sense, this activity is related to the physiological activity or the activity of the physiological system which produces a particular bio signal. The Hjorth activity (*HA*) is defined as,

$$HA = var(x(t))$$

where, *var* is the variance and $x(t)$ is the biosignal.

2.4.2 Hjorth Mobility

The average frequency of a bio signal is described by the Hjorth mobility. The mobility provides information about the speed of the physiological process. The Hjorth mobility is given by,

$$\text{Mobility} = \sqrt{\frac{\text{var}(x'(t))}{Var(x(t))}}$$

2.4.3 Hjorth Complexity

The Hjorth complexity describes the variability of the bio signal under analysis. The complexity of the given bio signal refers to the similarity of the bio signal to a sinusoidal wave. If the given signal is a pure sine curve, then its complexity is equal to 1.

The Hjorth complexity is given by,

$$\text{Complexity} = \frac{mobility(x'(t))}{mobility(x(t))}.$$

There are several studies in which Hjorth information has been successfully utilized for analysis of normal and abnormal biosignals. In one study by Alagumariappan et al., (2020), it is presented that even the changes in the diameter of the surface electrodes utilized for acquisition of biosignals can lead to changes in the Hjorth information of such signals. It was seen that average Hjorth activity, mobility and complexity of electrogastrograms acquired using surface electrodes with contact diameters of 16mm and 19mm was found to be significantly different (Alagumariappan et al., 2020) as presented in Table 2.1.

2.5 BIOSIGNALS AND CHAOS

The physiological system exhibits chaotic properties (Klonowski, 2009) and the dynamics associated with biological systems are highly nonlinear (Savi, 2005; Goldbeter, 2002). In most of the cases, health states are regarded as chaotic since these systems are able to well respond to perturbations. However, in systems with

TABLE 2.1
The Hjorth Information of Electrogastrograms Recorded Using Electrodes With Different Contact Diameters

Hjorth information (Average)	Contact diameter 16mm	Contact diameter 19mm
Activity	0.0148	0.0359
Mobility	0.0272	0.0526
Complexity	1.2351	1.3724

diseased states, there is a loss of flexibility and hence such systems may not be able to adapt or respond to external perturbations (Fisher, 1993). Several studies have demonstrated the importance of analysing the Lyapunov exponents and Hurst exponents for chaotic characterization of bio-signals (Das et al. 2002; Bradley, 1999). Fukunaga et al. (2000) have demonstrated that electrogastrograms can exhibit chaotic characteristics and the Lyapunov exponents can be utilized to quantify the effects of stress in analysis of electrogastrograms. Iasemidis et al., (2003) have developed an adaptive epileptic seizure prediction system based on chaotic analysis of EEG signals. Eidukaitis et al., (2004) have quantified the changes in the chaotic element of the cardiac rhythm at different sleep stages in healthy subjects of both sexes. Jovic and Bogunovic (2007) have applied chaos theory for ECG feature extraction. Padmanabhan and Puthusserypady, (2004) presented a systematic characterization of the EMG signals from leg muscles, using a nonlinear chaotic approach and reported that the signals were nonlinear and short-term stationary. Mengi et al., (2001) reported that EMG obeys a certain nonlinear deterministic law and is different from noise. Also, the estimation of chaos in bio-signals is useful for analysing the mechano-electric effects in the physiological system (Fukunaga et al., 2000).

To demonstrate the chaotic nature of electromyograms and the usefulness of chaotic analysis in differentiating normal and abnormal biosignals, the results of the chaotic analysis performed on 20 normal, 20 myopathic and 20 ALS EMG signals collected from the EMGlab opensource database is presented. The calculated maximum Lyapunov exponents of the collected signals are reported in Table 2.2. It is seen that there all the exponents are positive stating that the signals exhibit chaotic behaviour. Further, Figure 2.10 shows the variations in the maximum Lyapunov exponents of normal, myopathy and ALS signals. It is seen that the mean maximum Lyapunov exponent in the normal EMG signals is higher when compared to that of the other two cases.

Figures 2.11 to 2.16 show the variation of the Hurst exponents of normal and myopathic electromyograms, estimated using various methods such as the residuals of regression method, Higuchi's method, difference variance method, modified periodogram method, aggregate variance method and absolute moment method, correlated with the mean of the signals. Since the signal mean of EMG signals well correlates to the mean muscle force, the mean is taken as a good descriptor of the physiology of the muscles. Results demonstrate that that there are distinct variations between the normal and myopathic electromyograms in terms of their Hurst exponents and their correlation with the mean muscle forces. Further, the values of the Hurst exponents also vary with respect to the methods used.

The correlation of the Hurst exponents of normal and myopathic electromyograms estimated using various methods such as the residuals of regression method, Higuchi's method, difference variance method, modified periodogram method, aggregate variance method and absolute moment method, with the descriptive statistics of the EMG signals is presented in Table 2.3. It is seen that there are high degrees of correlation between the Hurst exponents and the statistical features. Further, it is found that the Hurst exponents estimated using the difference variance method and the modified periodogram method is of high statistical significance ($p < 0.001$) which denotes that these features can distinctively differentiate normal and myopathic electromyograms.

TABLE 2.2
The Maximum Lyapunov Exponent of Normal, Myopathy and ALS Electromyograms

	Maximum Lyapunov exponent		
Case	**Normal**	**Myopathy**	**ALS**
1	0.0053	0.0049	0.0019
2	0.0055	0.0050	0.0033
3	0.0061	0.0047	0.0047
4	0.0059	0.0051	0.0024
5	0.0052	0.0038	0.0033
6	0.0063	0.0039	0.0042
7	0.0051	0.0036	0.0040
8	0.0076	0.0038	0.0053
9	0.0054	0.0033	0.0049
10	0.0053	0.0040	0.0041
11	0.0056	0.0044	0.0045
12	0.0053	0.0053	0.0039
13	0.0051	0.0055	0.0044
14	0.0074	0.0053	0.0036
15	0.0043	0.0052	0.0051
16	0.0052	0.0047	0.0045
17	0.0054	0.0044	0.0037
18	0.0049	0.0044	0.0038
19	0.0052	0.003	0.0038
20	0.0061	0.0041	0.0046

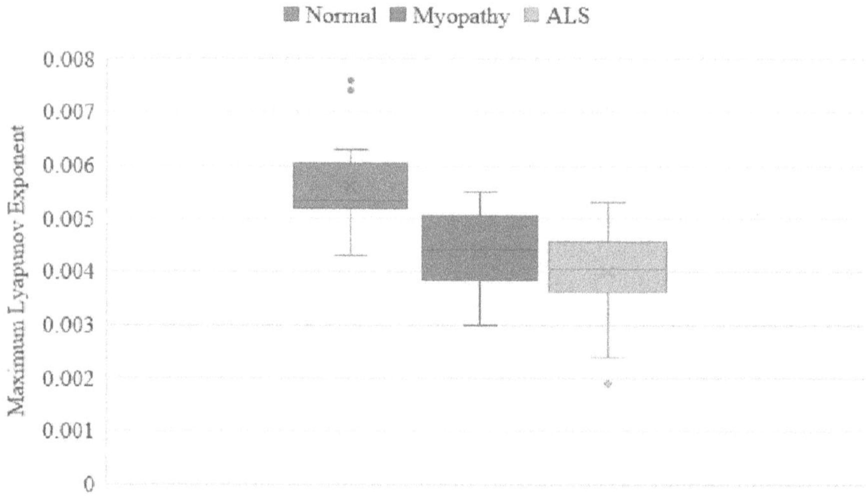

FIGURE 2.10 The variation in the maximum Lyapunov exponents of normal, myopathic and ALS EMG signals

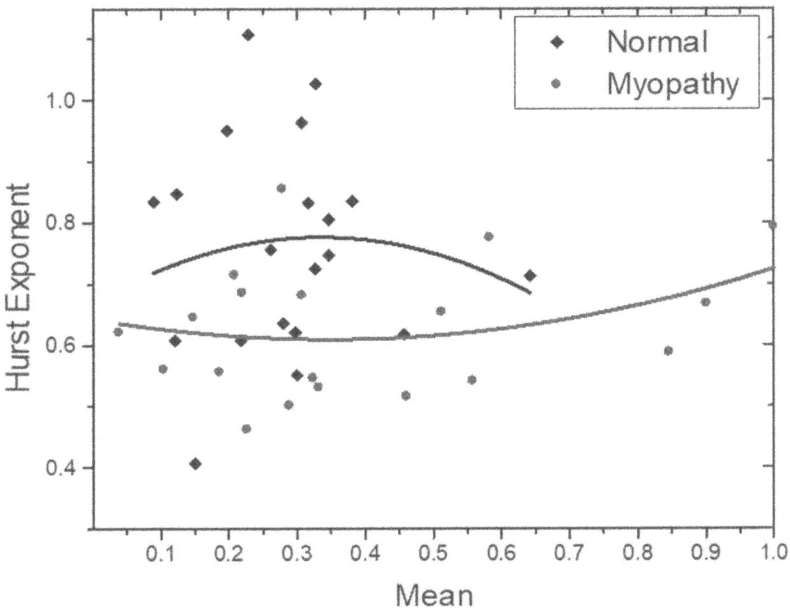

FIGURE 2.11 The variation of Hurst exponents of normal and myopathic EMG signals, calculated using the residuals of regression method, shown as a function of the mean of the signals

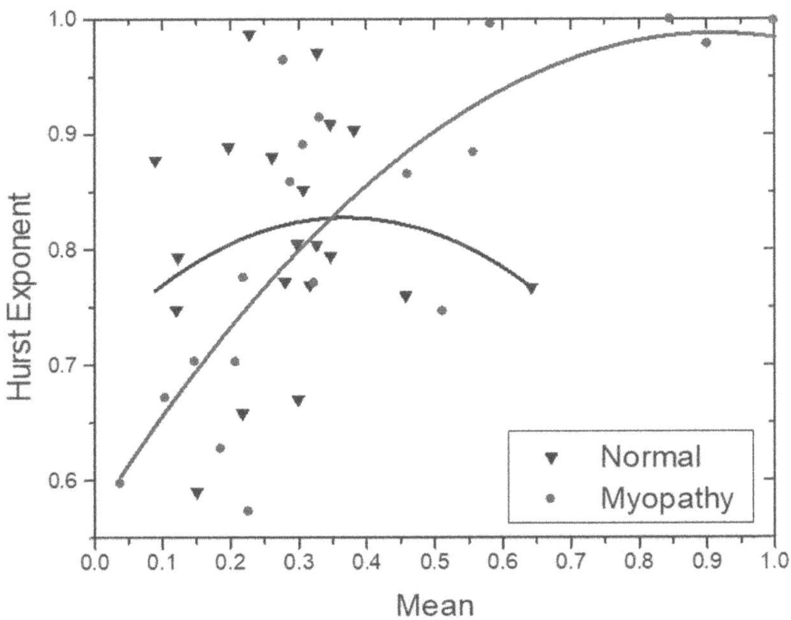

FIGURE 2.12 The variation of Hurst exponents of normal and myopathic EMG signals, calculated using the Higuchi's method, shown as a function of the mean of the signals

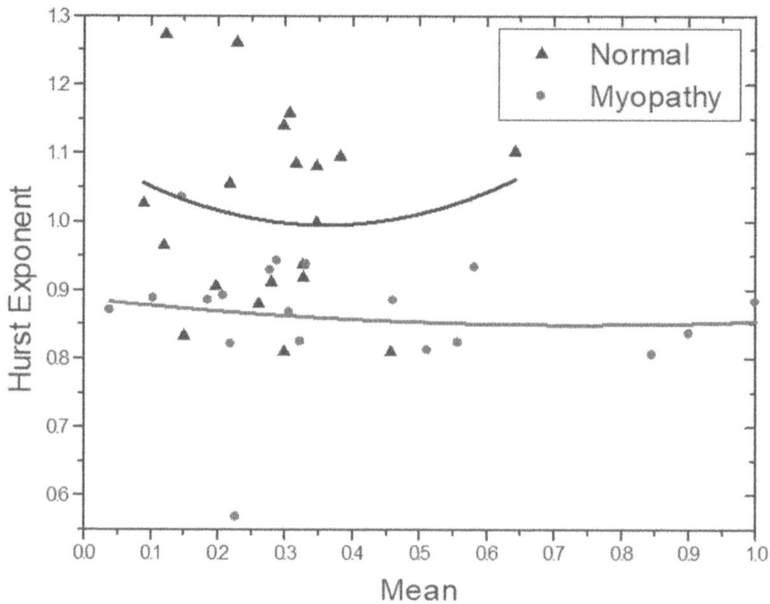

FIGURE 2.13 The variation of Hurst exponents of normal and myopathic EMG signals, calculated using the difference variance method, shown as a function of the mean of the signals

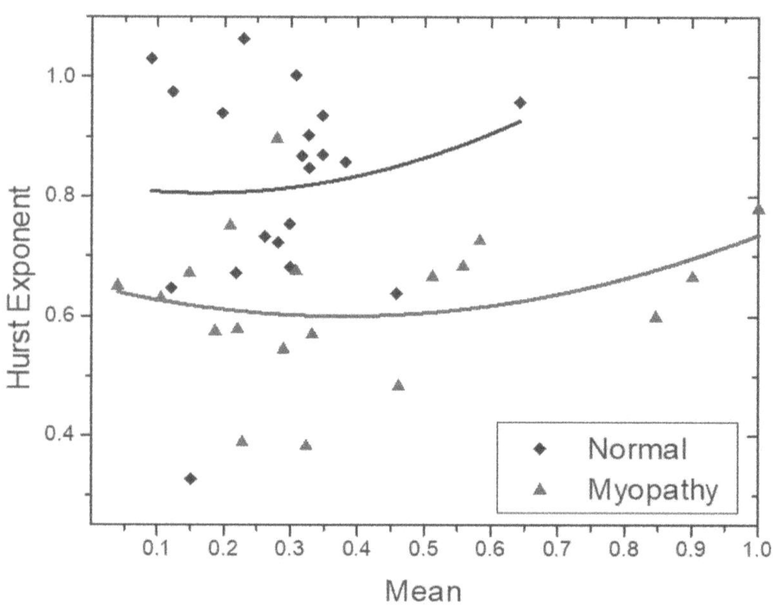

FIGURE 2.14 The variation of Hurst exponents of normal and myopathic EMG signals, calculated using the modified periodogram method, shown as a function of the mean of the signals

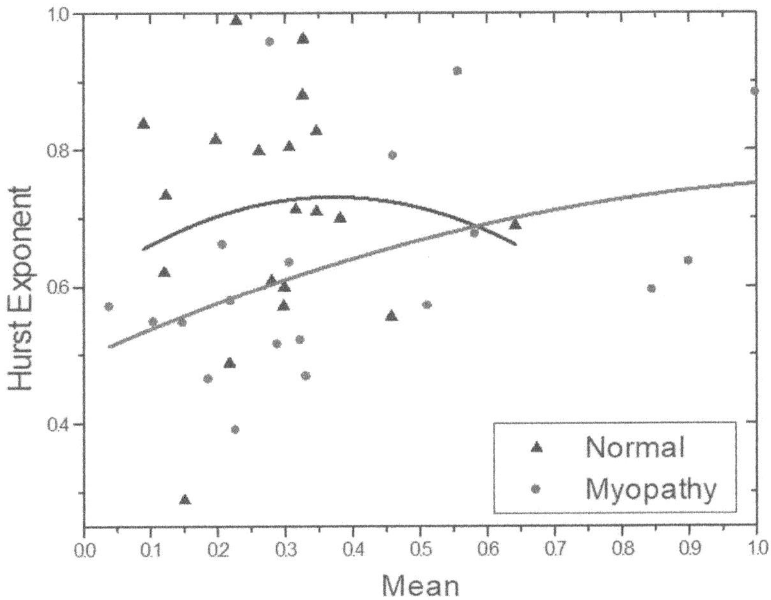

FIGURE 2.15 The variation of Hurst exponents of normal and myopathic EMG signals, calculated using the aggregate variance method, shown as a function of the mean of the signals

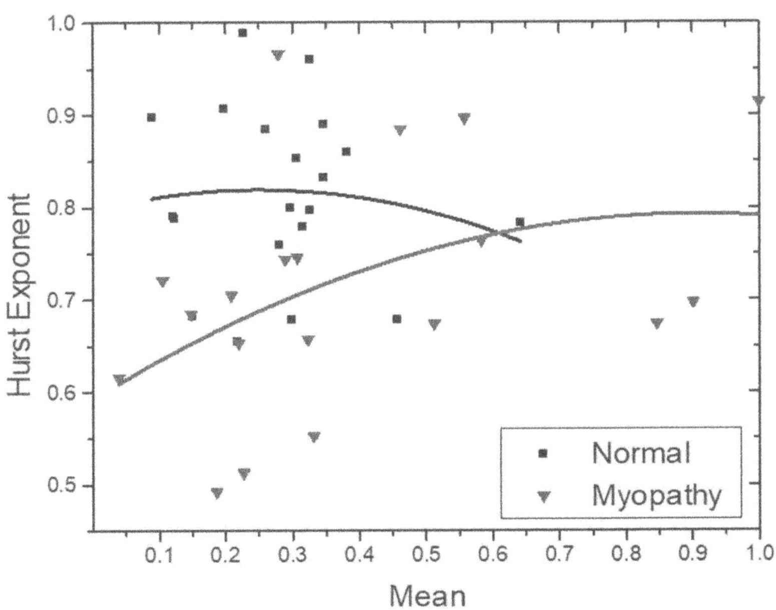

FIGURE 2.16 The variation of Hurst exponents of normal and myopathic EMG signals, calculated using the absolute moment method, shown as a function of the mean of the signals

TABLE 2.3
The Correlation of the Hurst Exponents Calculated Using Different Methods With the Descriptive Statistics of Normal and Myopathic Electromyograms Along With the Statistical Significance

			Descriptive Statistics					
		Diagnosis	**Mean**	**Median**	**Standard Deviation**	**Minimum Value**	**Maximum Value**	**Significance Value (p)**
Hurst Exponent	Residuals of regression method	Normal	0.14	0.50	0.37	0.42	**0.56**	0.0101
		Myopathy	0.31	0.33	0.20	0.24	0.31	
	Higuchi's method	Normal	0.20	**0.50**	**0.53**	0.46	**0.61**	0.906
		Myopathy	0.81	0.71	0.52	0.54	0.43	
	Difference Variance method	Normal	0.15	0.41	0.33	0.28	0.34	**0.00045**
		Myopathy	0.10	0.16	0.47	**0.70**	**0.76**	
	Modified periodogram method	Normal	0.15	**0.60**	0.20	**0.62**	**0.55**	**0.00191**
		Myopathy	0.30	0.24	0.16	0.31	0.31	
	Aggregate variance method	Normal	0.15	**0.53**	0.31	0.48	**0.51**	0.0996
		Myopathy	0.44	0.35	0.18	0.36	0.33	
	Absolute moment method	Normal	0.13	**0.50**	**0.50**	0.29	**0.50**	**0.0034**
		Myopathy	0.42	0.34	0.19	0.42	0.43	

REFERENCES

Ahmad, S. A., & Chappell, P. H. (2008). Moving approximate entropy applied to surface electromyographic signals. *Biomedical Signal Processing and Control*, 3(*1*), 88–93.

Ahsan, M. R., Ibrahimy, M. I., & Khalifa, O. O. (2009). EMG signal classification for human computer interaction: a review. *European Journal of Scientific Research*, 33(*3*), 480–501.

Alagumariappan, P., Krishnamurthy, K., & Jawahar, P. M. (2020). Selection of surface electrodes for electrogastrography and analysis of normal and abnormal electrogastrograms using Information. *International Journal of Biomedical Engineering and Technology*, 32(*4*), 317–330.

Ambikapathy, B., & Krishnamurthy, K. (2018). Analysis of electromyograms recorded using invasive and noninvasive electrodes: a study based on entropy and Lyapunov exponents estimated using artificial neural networks. *Journal of Ambient Intelligence and Humanized Computing*, 1–9.

Ambikapathy, B., Kirshnamurthy, K., & Venkatesan, R. (2018). Assessment of electromyograms using genetic algorithm and artificial neural networks. *Evolutionary Intelligence*, 1–11.

Azami, H., Rostaghi, M., Abásolo, D., & Escudero, J. (2017). Refined composite multiscale dispersion entropy and its application to biomedical signals. *IEEE Transactions on Biomedical Engineering*, 64(*12*), 2872–2879.

Bakiya, A., & Kamalanand, K. (2018). Information analysis on electromyograms acquired using monopolar needle, concentric needle and surface electrodes. In *2018 International Conference on Recent Trends in Electrical, Control and Communication (RTECC)* (pp. 240–244). IEEE.

Bakiya, A., Kamalanand, K., Rajinikanth, V., Nayak, R. S., & Kadry, S. (2018). Deep neural network assisted diagnosis of time-frequency transformed electromyograms. *Multimedia Tools and Applications,* 1–17.

Boashash, B. (2015). *Time-Frequency Signal Analysis and Processing: A Comprehensive Reference*. Academic Press.

Bradley, E. (1999). Time-series analysis. *Intelligent Data Analysis: An Introduction. Springer.*

Brooks, D. R., Wiley, E. O., & Brooks, D. R. (1988). *Evolution as Entropy.* University of Chicago Press.

Cacioppo, J. T., & Petty, R. E. (1981). Electromyograms as measures of extent and affectivity of information processing. *American Psychologist*, 36(*5*), 441.

Carlen, E. A., Carvalho, M. C., Roux, J. L., Loss, M., & Villani, C. (2008). Entropy and chaos in the kac model. *arXiv preprint arXiv:0808*.3192.

Castiglioni, P., Piskorski, J., Kośmider, M., Guzik, P., Rampichini, E., & Merati, S., G. (2013). Assessing sample entropy of physiological signals by the norm component matrix algorithm: Application on muscular signals during isometric contraction. In *2013 35th Annual International Conference of the IEEE Engineering in Medicine and Biology Society (EMBC)* (pp. 5053–5056). IEEE.

Cerf, N. J., & Adami, C. (1997). Negative entropy and information in quantum mechanics. *Physical Review Letters*, 79(*26*), 5194.

Chen, W., Wang, Z., Xie, H., & Yu, W. (2007). Characterization of surface EMG signal based on fuzzy entropy. *IEEE Transactions on neural systems and rehabilitation engineering*, 15(2), 266–272.

Damaševičius, R., Maskeliūnas, R., Woźniak, M., & Połap, D. (2018). Visualization of physiologic signals based on Hjorth parameters and Gramian angular fields. In *2018 IEEE 16th World Symposium on Applied Machine Intelligence and Informatics (SAMI)* (pp. 000091–000096). IEEE.

Das, A., Das, P., & Roy, A. B. (2002). Applicability of Lyapunov exponent in EEG data analysis. *Complexity International*, 9(das01), 1–8.

Dickhaus, H., & Heinrich, H. (1996). Classifying biosignals with wavelet networks [a method for noninvasive diagnosis]. *IEEE Engineering in Medicine and Biology Magazine*, 15(*5*), 103–111.

Dietz, V., Schmidtbleicher, D., & Noth, J. (1979). Neuronal mechanisms of human locomotion. *Journal of Neurophysiology*, 42(*5*), 1212–1222.

Eidukaitis, A., Varoneckas, G., & Žemaityteė, D. (2004). Application of chaos theory in analyzing the cardiac rhythm in healthy subjects at different sleep stages. *Human Physiology*, 30(*5*), 551–555.

EMGlab: http://www.emglab.net/

Escabí, M. (2012). Biosignal Processing. In *Introduction to Biomedical Engineering* (pp. 667–746). Academic Press.

Escabí, M. A. (2005). Biosignal Processing. In *Introduction to Biomedical Engineering* (pp. 549–625). Academic Press.

Fisher, G. V. (1993). An introduction to chaos theory and some haematological applications. *Comparative Haematology International*, 3(*1*), 43–51.

Fukunaga, M., Arita, S., Ishino, S., & Nakai, Y. (2000). Quantitative analysis of gastric electric stress response with chaos theory. *International Journal of Biomedical Soft Computing and Human Sciences: the official journal of the Biomedical Fuzzy Systems Association*, 5(2), 59–64.

Gil, L. M., Nunes, T. P., Silva, F. H., Faria, A. C., & Melo, P. L. (2010). Analysis of human tremor in patients with Parkinson disease using entropy measures of signal complexity. In *2010 Annual International Conference of the IEEE Engineering in Medicine and Biology* (pp. 2786–2789). IEEE.

Goldbeter, A. (2002). Computational approaches to cellular rhythms. *Nature*, 420(*6912*), 238–245.

Gratton, G. (2007). Biosignal processing.

Gray, R. M. (2011). *Entropy and Information Theory*. Springer Science & Business Media.

Hamida, S. T. B., Ahmed, B., & Penzel, T. (2015). A novel insomnia identification method based on Hjorth parameters. In *2015 IEEE International Symposium on Signal Processing and Information Technology (ISSPIT)* (pp. 548–552). IEEE.

Harris, F. J. (1987). Time domain signal processing with the DFT. In *Handbook of Digital Signal Processing* (pp. 633–699). Academic Press.

Iasemidis, L. D., Shiau, D. S., Chaovalitwongse, W., Sackellares, J. C., Pardalos, P. M., Principe, J. C., & Tsakalis, K. (2003). Adaptive epileptic seizure prediction system. *IEEE Transactions on Biomedical Engineering*, 50(*5*), 616–627.

Javadpour, A., & Mohammadi, A. (2015). Implementing a smart method to eliminate artifacts of vital signals. *Journal of Biomedical Physics & Engineering*, 5(*4*), 199.

Jovic, A., & Bogunovic, N. (2007). Feature extraction for ECG time-series mining based on chaos theory. In *2007 29th International Conference on Information Technology Interfaces* (pp. 63–68). IEEE.

Klonowski, W. (2009). Everything you wanted to ask about EEG but were afraid to get the right answer. *Nonlinear Biomedical Physics*, 3(*1*), 1–5.

Kugelberg, E. (1947). Electromyograms in muscular disorders. *Journal of Neurology, Neurosurgery, and Psychiatry*, 10(*3*), 122.

Levkov, C. L. (1988). Amplification of biosignals by body potential driving. Analysis of the circuit performance. *Medical and Biological Engineering and Computing*, 26(*4*), 389.

Liang, H., Bronzino, J. D., & Peterson, D. R. (Eds.). (2012). *Biosignal Processing: Principles and Practices*. CRC Press.

Lotte, F., Congedo, M., Lécuyer, A., Lamarche, F., & Arnaldi, B. (2007). A review of classification algorithms for EEG-based brain–computer interfaces. *Journal of Neural Engineering*, 4(2), R1.

Medved, V. (2000). *Measurement of Human Locomotion*. CRC press.
Mengi, Y., Liu, B., & Liu, Y. (2001). A comprehensive nonlinear analysis of electromyogram. In *2001 Conference Proceedings of the 23rd Annual International Conference of the IEEE Engineering in Medicine and Biology Society* (Vol. 2, pp. 1078–1081). IEEE.
Naït-Ali, A. (Ed.). (2009). *Advanced Biosignal Processing*. Springer Science & Business Media.
Oh, S. H., Lee, Y. R., & Kim, H. N. (2014). A novel EEG feature extraction method using Hjorth parameter. *International Journal of Electronics and Electrical Engineering*, 2(2), 106–110.
Padmanabhan, P., & Puthusserypady, S. (2004). Nonlinear analysis of EMG signals-a chaotic approach. In *The 26th Annual International Conference of the IEEE Engineering in Medicine and Biology Society* (Vol. 1, pp. 608–611). IEEE.
Pham, T. D. (2017). Time-shift multiscale entropy analysis of physiological signals. *Entropy*, 19(*6*), 257.
PhysioBank Database: https://archive.physionet.org/physiobank/
Ren, P., Zhao, W., Zhao, Z., Bringas-Vega, M. L., Valdes-Sosa, P. A., & Kendrick, K. M. (2015). Analysis of gait rhythm fluctuations for neurodegenerative diseases by phase synchronization and conditional entropy. *IEEE Transactions on Neural Systems and Rehabilitation Engineering*, 24(*2*), 291–299.
Savi, M. A. (2005). Chaos and order in biomedical rhythms. *Journal of the Brazilian Society of Mechanical Sciences and Engineering*, 27(2), 157–169.
Sejdić, E., Lowry, K. A., Bellanca, J., Redfern, M. S., & Brach, J. S. (2013). A comprehensive assessment of gait accelerometry signals in time, frequency and time-frequency domains. *IEEE Transactions on Neural Systems and Rehabilitation Engineering*, 22(*3*), 603–612.
Semmlow, J. (2017). *Circuits, Signals and Systems for Bioengineers: A MATLAB-Based Introduction*. Academic Press.
Semmlow, J. L., & Griffel, B. (2014). *Biosignal and Medical Image Processing*. CRC press.
Shiavi, R., Frigo, C., & Pedotti, A. (1998). Electromyographic signals during gait: criteria for envelope filtering and number of strides. *Medical and Biological Engineering and Computing*, 36(2), 171–178.
Singh, Y. N., Singh, S. K., & Ray, A. K. (2012). Bioelectrical signals as emerging biometrics: issues and challenges. *ISRN Signal Processing.*
Srinivasan, V., Eswaran, C., & Sriraam, N. (2007). Approximate entropy-based epileptic EEG detection using artificial neural networks. *IEEE Transactions on Information Technology in Biomedicine*, 11(*3*), 288–295.
Supratak, A., Wu, C., Dong, H., Sun, K., & Guo, Y. (2016). Survey on feature extraction and applications of biosignals. In *Machine Learning for Health Informatics* (pp. 161). Springer.
Taga, G. (1995). A model of the neuro-musculo-skeletal system for human locomotion. *Biological cybernetics*, 73(*2*), 97–111.
Tamil, E. M., Bashar, N. S., Idris, M. Y. I., & Tamil, A. M. (2008). A review on feature extraction & classification techniques for biosignal processing (part iii: Electromyogram). In *4th Kuala Lumpur International Conference on Biomedical Engineering 2008* (pp. 117–121). Springer, Berlin, Heidelberg.
Toker, D., Sommer, F. T., & D'Esposito, M. (2020). A simple method for detecting chaos in nature. *Communications Biology*, 3(*1*), 1–13.
Tranquillo, J. V. (2013). Biomedical signals and systems. *Synthesis Lectures on Biomedical Engineering*, 8(*3*), 1–233.
Van Bemmel, J. H., Sato, S., Kazuo, Y., & Saranummi, N. (1997). Biosignal interpretation. *Methods of Information in Medicine*, 36(04/05), 235–236.

Xue, F., Wang, C. G., & Mu, F. (2011). Genetic and ant colony collaborative optimization algorithm based on information entropy and chaos theory. *Control and Decision*, 26(*1*), 44–48.

Zhang, X. D. (2017). Entropy for the complexity of physiological signal dynamics. In *Healthcare and Big Data Management* (pp. 39). Springer.

3 Need for Medical Imaging and Its Modalities

The rapid development in modern science and technology supports the people with an improved living ambience. The superior livelihood assists the persons to use an ample services; including the state of the art medical services with field level and remote monitoring facilities. Further, a considerable amount of vaccination and preventive medicine helped to reduce the happening of infectious and transmissible diseases. The sophisticated treatment facilities in multi-specialty hospitals also maintain the early detection of the disease and treatment implementation using improved monitoring facilities. Moreover, scheduled health checkups are commonly suggested by the doctor; who helps to recognize and cure a number of acute diseases in its early phase.

Even though substantial methods are engaged to prevent and heal the diseases in human; the occurrence rate of communicable and non-communicable syndromes are rapidly growing due to a variety of reasons, such as gender, age, race, etc. To maintain the premature analysis and treatment execution for the disease; a number of diagnostic trial are proposed and executed in various disease diagnostic centres and clinics. The medical images registered by means of a preferred modality gives essential insight concerning the disease to be identified and based on this information; the doctor would plan for the handling procedures to be executed to control/ cure the disease (Chaki and Dey, 2020; Dougherty, 1994; Priya and Srinivasan, 2015; Bhandary et al., 2020).

In recent years, medical images recorded with a suitable technique play a vital role in hospitals. The medical imagining procedures along with a suitable computer algorithm will help to diagnose the orientation and the infection rate with better accuracy and this information is to be accounted by the doctor, when a visual assessment and confirmation. The choice of an appropriate imaging modality depends mainly on the infection to be analysed, the organ to be examined and expertise of the doctor who suggests the imaging procedure. The medical images can be registered using various methods ranging from the digital camera to the radiation supported imaging. The medical grade images recorded may be: (i) Greyscale or RGB scale and (ii) Two-dimensional (2D) or 3D and during the automated assessment a chosen pre-processing and post-processing technique can be implemented to extract the information. Most of the recent imaging procedures are supervised by the computers and hence getting the digital form of the image is quite simple and the attained digital images can be processed and stored easily with appropriate digital memory devices.

This chapter presents the overview of disease screening methods for few chosen domains, such as osteoporosis, retinal health, skin cancer, disease in lungs, brain abnormality, and breast abnormality. A brief overview of the imaging modalities and its assessment technique is presented with suitable examples. Further, this chapter also outlines the role of the computer supported schemes executed to improve the detection accuracy for a range of clinical images.

3.1 DISEASE IN HUMAN ORGANS

In the current scenario, any acute or infectious disuse in human is a vital medical emergency and all the possible methodologies are to be executed during the diagnosis, treatment planning and execution. During the treatment execution, the patient can be admitted and monitored in hospital level or the patient can be monitored with routine health checkups as suggested by the doctor. A variety of medical protocols are followed during the disease detection in humans, which includes a visual check, signal-assisted diagnosis and image-assisted diagnosis and the choice of these procedures depends on the nature of the disease and the experience of the doctor.

Diseases in external body organs can be detected and treated easily compared to the internal organs due to its accessibility and the visual check based initial assessment works well during the disease screening procedures executed for eyes, skin and breast. Disease in internal organs is more acute and untreated disease will lead to temporary or permanent disability and some time it may lead to death. Visual check cannot be implemented for the internal organ inspections; hence suitable medical imaging methods are recommended and implemented to record the infected section of the organ for the diagnosis and treatment.

The recent development in medical imagining procedure helped to diagnose the disease in internal organs using a chosen imaging modalities. The advancement in imaging procedures helped to capture the picture of the organ in greyscale or RGB form and the doctor will assess these images using a suitable methodology to confirm the disease. The recorded images can also be used to track the sequence of the illness with reverence to the time. Recognition of the illness in its early stage is very essential to plan for the suitable treatment. A scheduled body screening will help to identify a number of diseases in its premature phase, even though the symptoms are absent. Hence, in recent years, a number of medical protocols are proposed and implemented to ensure the normal functioning of the body parts and these procedures also helped in detecting the various acute diseases in its early phase.

The overview of the clinical level analytical methods of the disease in various human organs is presented in this division with suitable examples.

Figure 3.1 depicts the different stages concerned in the preliminary checks by a doctor; when an infected patient approaches. When the patient approach a doctor after recognizing the possible disease symptom; the doctor will execute all the initial checks as per the medical etiquette; which comprises the universal verification, such

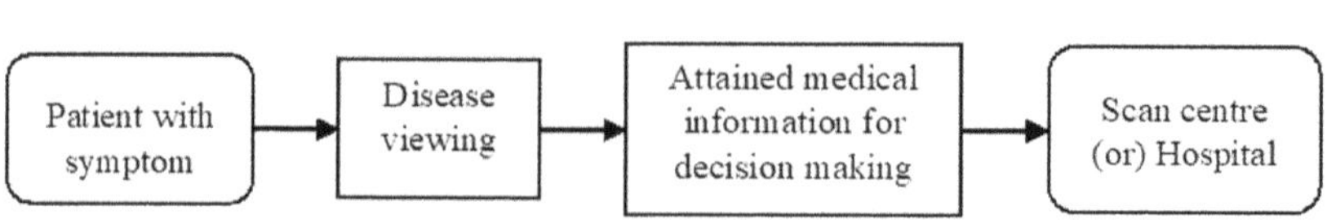

FIGURE 3.1 Preliminary check and suggestion by a doctor

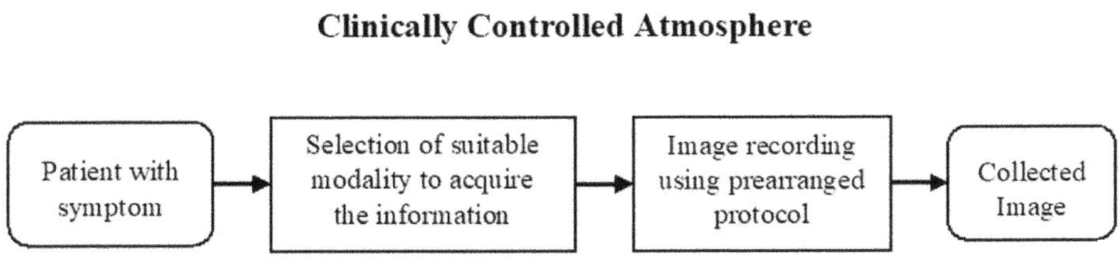

FIGURE 3.2 Implementation of recommended protocol to collect the disease information

as gender, age, weight, earlier illness history, duration and the severity of symptoms felt by the patient, heart rate, temperature check and other recommended checks to recognize the reason and severity of the disease. If the disease is associated with an internal organ, along with the personal check; the doctor also will suggest a clinical check to reach essential information regarding the disease. After carefully analysing the medical report, the doctor will plan for a suitable action to control/cure the illness.

Figure 3.2 presents the different stages associated in recording of infection in vital internal organ with the recommended imaging modality. The illness in the interior organ is primarily appraised by a doctor and for additional evaluation; the picture of the organ is to be recorded using a selected modality. To enhance the quality and also to maintain the privacy, the image recording process is to be executed in a controlled setting and all the approved etiquette is to be followed throughout the process in order to avoid the ethical and legal issues. After collecting the picture, the preliminary appraisal is performed in the scan/imaging hub and the recorded picture along with the forecast is then submitted for the doctor for the additional assessment. The doctor will scrutinize the picture and the report and based on this inspection, a conclusion regarding the orientation, reason and severity of the disease will be computed and essential treatment procedure is suggested and implemented.

Figure 3.3 depicts the frequent picture assessment scheme employed to examine the medical images collected with a preferred modality. After getting the picture from a patient, the raw image experience a variety of pre-processing operations based on the need; some of the regularly considered image pre-processing techniques are: (i) image orientation adjustment, (ii) resizing, (iii) filtering, (iv) contrast enhancement, etc. After the pre-processing, a preferred post-processing practice is then executed to extract the necessary division or the features from the image; which then support in the diagnosis of the disease using dedicated computerized software.

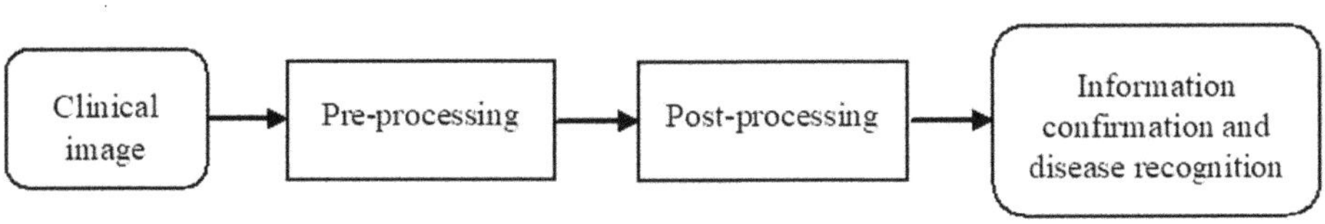

FIGURE 3.3 Image evaluation procedure to extract the disease information

Due to its medical significance, a considerable amount of semi-automated and automated illness recognition schemes are proposed by the researchers to identify a variety of diseases. The disease assessment schemes will act as the supporting systems for the doctor who takes the conclusion during the treatment execution.

The forthcoming sub-sections of this chapter presents the essential information on a variety of imaging modalities considered to record the images in greyscale or RGB scale using a chosen technique. The presented medical images in these chapters are collected from the well-known benchmark image datasets existing in the literature. A short discussion about each image is presented and the available assessment procedures for these images are also discussed in brief.

3.2 NEED FOR MEDICAL IMAGING TECHNIQUES

Imaging procedures are widely adopted in medical domain to evaluate the abnormality in human physiology and in general; a variety of medical image acquiring techniques are existing in the literature to record in essential information from cell-level to organ-level (Dey et al., 2019; Rajinikanth et al., 2020; Priya et al., 2014). Based on the need, it is essential to choose and implement a prescribed procedure, which helps in getting the essential information.

The invasive/non-invasive medical imaging practice considerably improved the medical field and due to its importance, still a considerable number of ongoing research works are performed to discover the new image registering and enhancing procedures. Compared to the invasive techniques, non-invasive techniques are widely adopted due to its simplicity and ease in execution. The present chapter discusses only the limited imaging procedures adopted to examine the various human parts, such as bone, eye, skin, lungs, brain and breast. Figure 3.4 presents the non-invasive imaging procedures adopted for the body parts and the disease which can be assessed with chosen imaging modalities

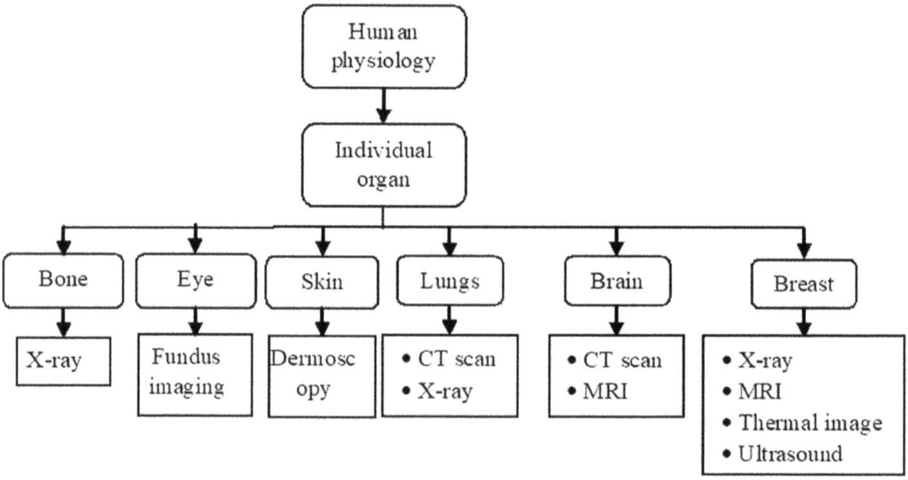

FIGURE 3.4 Imaging procedures considered to analyse the body organ

3.2.1 Examination of Bone

Bone is a rigid part in human physiology, which gives the shape and strength to the body. The normal property of the bone may be affected due to a variety of reasons, such as ageing, accident and the disease. The abnormality in bone due to accident is insignificant compared to the abnormality due to aging. Since, most of the elderly people may experience a bone disease called the osteoporosis, which may weaken the bone and may cause mild to serious health issues including the temporary/ permanent disability.

The osteoporosis may form porous-bone due to the mineral deficiency and if the disease is detected in its early phase; it is curable with a proper diet and medication. Normally, the bone sections are examined using the radiology assisted imaging technique called X-ray and a film based or digital x-ray images of the bone is evaluated by a radiologist and the orthopaedic specialist. Based on the evaluation outcome of the bone X-ray, possible treatment suggestion is taken.

The common procedure followed to examine the osteoporosis using the skeletal X-ray is depicted in Figure 3.5. When the patient experiences the symptom; then a clinical level assessment is to be done by a doctor and based on the suggestion, a skeletal X-ray is recorded and examined. The report attained from the skeletal X-ray is then considered o plan for an appropriate treatment.

Figure 3.6 presents the clinical grade skeletal X-ray collected from the XSITRAY database (Fathima et al., 2019; Fathima et al., 2020). This database is having the digital X-ray images of essential skeletal sections, such as spine, femur and clavicle sections and the previous research work on these images are considered to evaluate the Bone-Mineral-Density (BMD) (Chavan et al., 2020; McClung et al., 2014; Marshall et al., 1996).

The raw image attained from the clinics needs few pre-processing procedures, such as cropping the unwanted sections/image labels and it also needs the resizing (512x512x1 pixels) for the image normalization. After implementing the essential initial processing, the bone sections are enhanced using a chosen image processing technique and then its BMD is assessed.

If the existing level of the BMD is predicted using a suitable computerized algorithm, the report will be verified and the suggestions will be provided by the doctor. The possible treatment for the osteoporosis will include; exercise (to strengthen bone and surrounded muscles), nutrition (increasing calcium and vitamin D related supplement) and limiting smoking/alcohol intake (for selected people). The earlier research work also indicated that, if the BMD level is diagnosed with better accuracy, the effect of the osteoporosis can be completely cured. Further, this problem can also be stopped with the help of a scheduled image-assisted diagnosis.

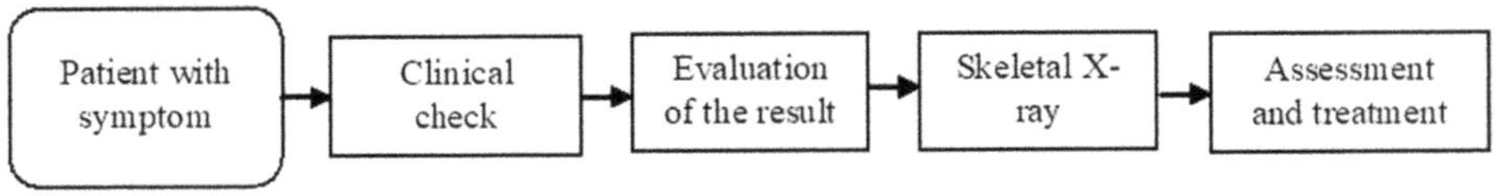

FIGURE 3.5 Recording of the bone X-ray for osteoporosis assessment

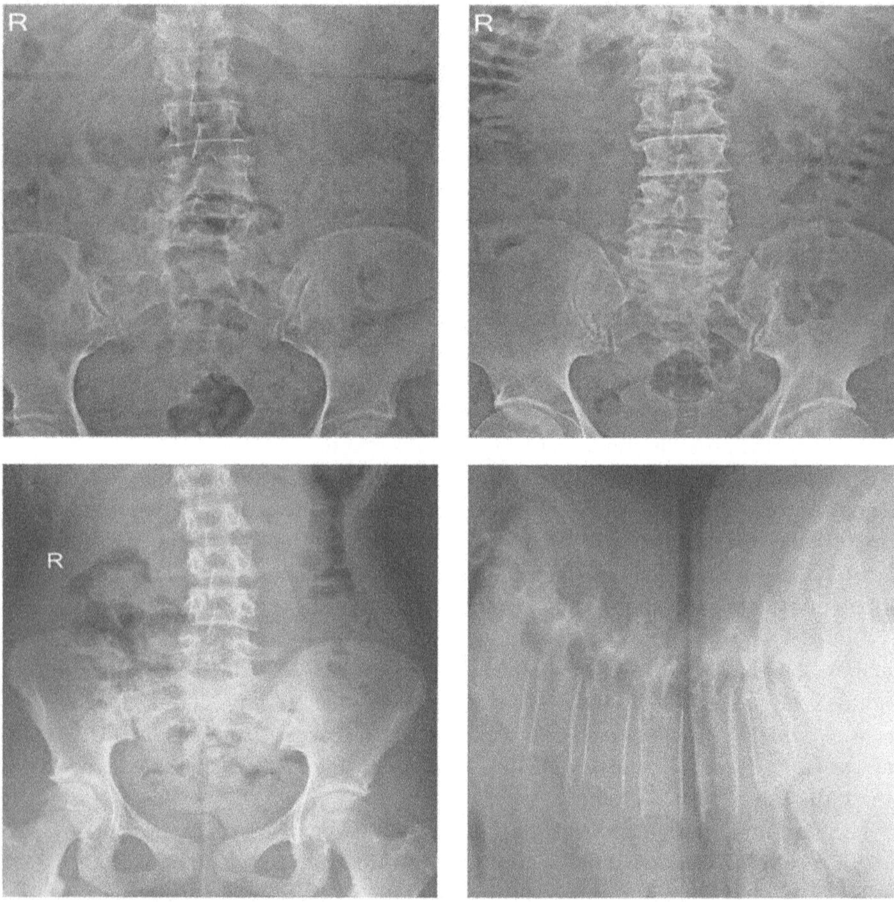

FIGURE 3.6 Clinical grade X-ray images considered to assess the BMD

3.2.2 Examination of Eye

The disease in eye arises due to a variety of reasons, such as ageing, accident, infection, etc. and the untreated eye disease will lead to the loss of vision. If the vision system is disturbed, then the decision-making process of the brain also will be severely affected. The eye disease is one of the common problems in humans and found globally irrespective of their race and gender. The illness in eye generally needs a personal check by a knowledgeable ophthalmologist and then an image guided assessment.

During the image supported assessment, a particular imaging scheme recorded with the fundus camera is used to analyse the retinal part for further evaluation. Fundus camera registers the retina, the neuro-sensory tissue in our eyes which decode the optical images into the electrical impulses for the brain. During image acquisition, the patient is allowed to be seated at the fundus camera with their chin positioned in a chin rest and their forehead against the imaging system.

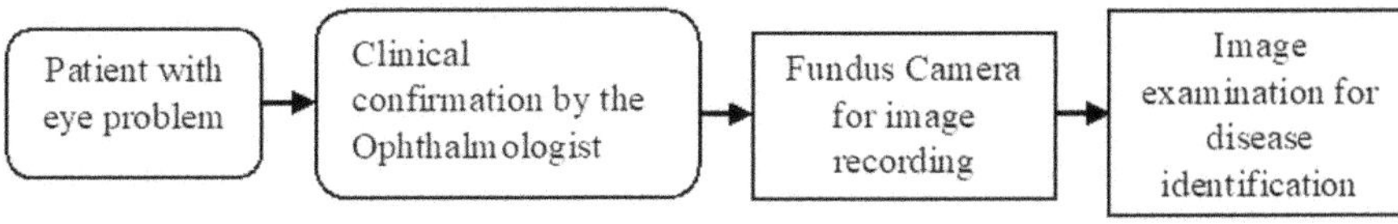

FIGURE 3.7 Clinical level screening practice executed to detect eye abnormality

An ophthalmologist focuses and line-up the fundus camera. A controlled light beam is then passed into the eye and the necessary picture is then recorded. The previous works in the literature confirms that, the fundus image supported practice can be used to notice a range of eye diseases. Figure 3.7 presents the protocol followed during the retinal image recording process and Figure 3.8 shows a typical fundus

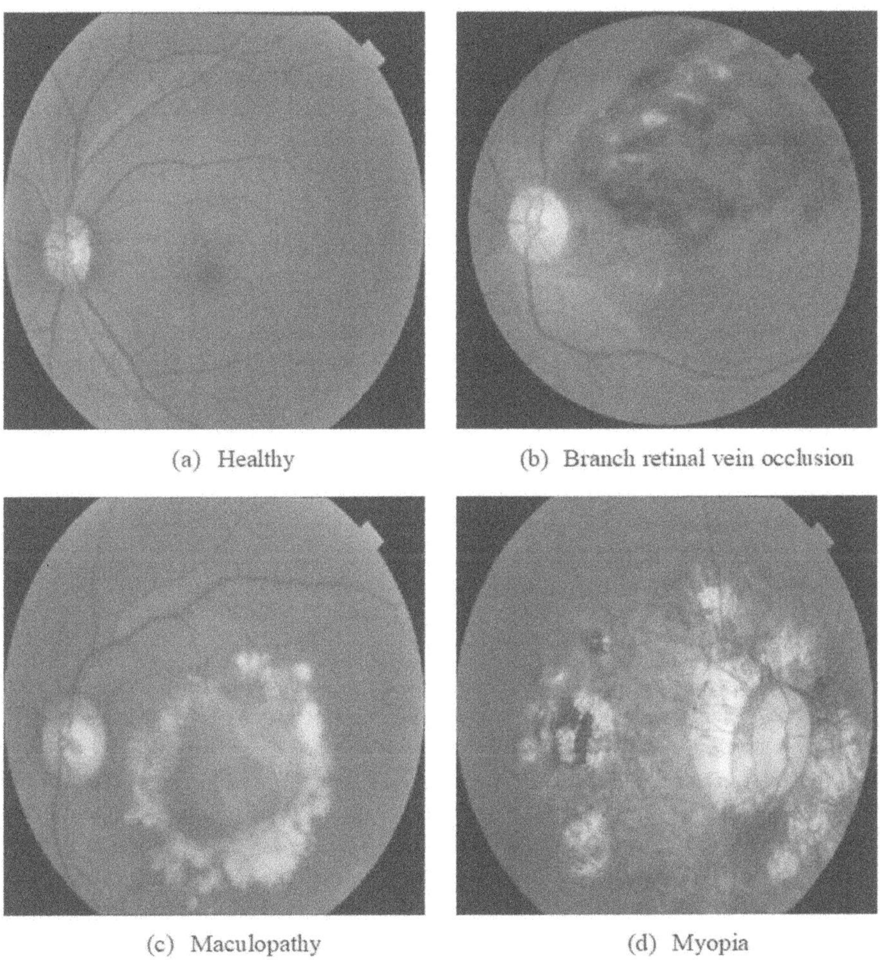

FIGURE 3.8 Sample fundus images of retinal for healthy and disease class

illustration collected from the benchmark retinal database of various classes. These images are then examined by an experienced ophthalmologist or a computer algorithm to assess the disease and this information is then considered to plan and execute the treatment to cure the eye disease (Shree et al., 2018; Shriranjani et al., 2018; Sudhan et al., 2017; Rajinikanth et al., 2020a).

3.2.3 Examination of Skin

The dangerous skin level disease is the skin cancer and it is one of the widespread cancers in humans mainly due to the high spotlight of the skin to Ultraviolet Light (UV) rays. When the pigment-producing cells called the melanocytes are exposed to the high-grade UV ray will boost the possibility of the skin melanoma in humans. The early identification of the melanoma is necessary to cure the illness using possible treatment methodologies, including the surgery. When the disease stage is acute, it will discharge the cancerous cells in the blood stream and hence the cancer cells will extend to other very important body parts and reduce the chances of the recovery of patient from death. The recognition of the melanoma in its early stage needs a self-verification followed by a screening by a practiced dermatologist. The dermatologist will distinguish the skin cancer by means of the regularly prescribed ABCDE rule, which helps to separate the moles from melanoma (Dey et al., 2018; Rajinikanth et al., 2019).

The ABCDE regulation assists to distinguish the skin cancer according to the following constraints (Rajinikanth et al., 2019a);

- Asymmetric: The ordinary moles are probably in circular shape and balanced, but one side of a cancerous mole is possibly to look different to the other surface.
- Border: The external surface is asymmetrical rather than smooth and may become visible tattered, uneven, or blurred.
- Color: Melanoma segment may tend to have inconsistent shades and colours, including black, brown, and tan.
- Diameter: Melanoma can cause a modified size in a mole.
- Evolving: Difference in a mole's exterior over weeks or months can be a sign of melanoma.

The medical stage recognition of the melanoma is achieved with the ABCDE rule with an assessment using the dermoscopy. The computerized dermoscopy will assist to record the doubtful skin sections for the future appraisal and the sample test images collected for the demonstration is presented in Figure 3.9. In Figure 3.9 (a) depicts the mole (nevus), Figure 3.9 (b) presents melanoma. When the skin abnormality is associated with the hair section, the automated assessment will become a problem and during the diagnosis, the evaluation along with the hair section may present false result when a hence a number of hair removal scheme is proposed and implemented to enhance the skin section during the dermoscopy image assessment. The earlier research on the skin melanoma can be accessed from (Kowsalya et al., 2018).

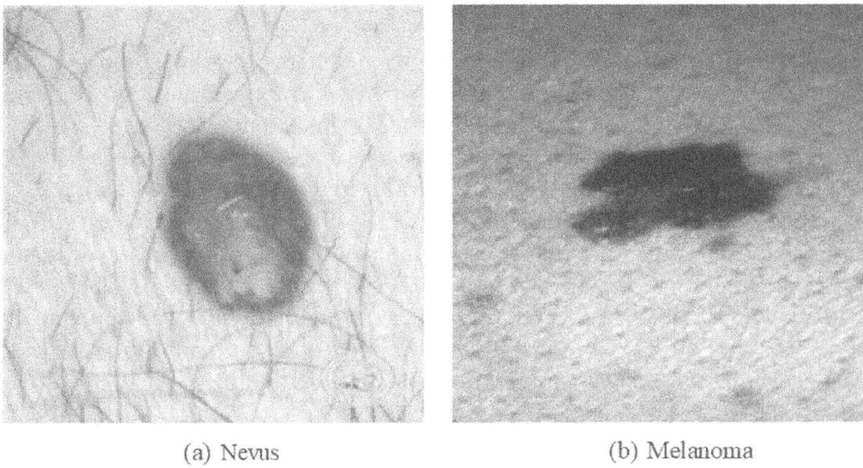

FIGURE 3.9 Sample dermoscopy images for skin abnormality assessment

The skin melanoma is one of the life threats in a variety of countries and infects a number of people every year. The clinical level identification of the melanoma includes the (i) Image based recognition and (ii) Biopsy assisted detection and substantiation. In the image supported analysis, the dermoscopy images are scrutinized by a doctor or a computer algorithm to verify the illness with the help of the parameters presents in ABCD rule. During the biopsy test, sample of the skin tissue are collected by means of the medical protocol and these tissues are tested in clinics to confirm the cancer and its stage. When the cancer is confirmed throughout the biopsy test, a surgery is suggested by the doctor to eliminate the infected skin part in order to stop the spreading of the disease. The skin melanoma diagnosis with picture-based techniques can be found in (Glaister, 2013; Rajinikanth et al., 2017; Nair et al., 2019).

Clinical level assessment of the skin-melanoma is presented in Figure 3.10. The general practice followed in diagnosing the skin level disease by means of the dermoscopy is depicted below. If the imaging procedure presents a suspicious result, then a biopsy is implemented to confirm the disease. If the skin cancer is confirmed, then the treatment is implemented to manage the spread of the cancer to other tissues and the contaminated skin segment is carefully removed by implementing the surgery.

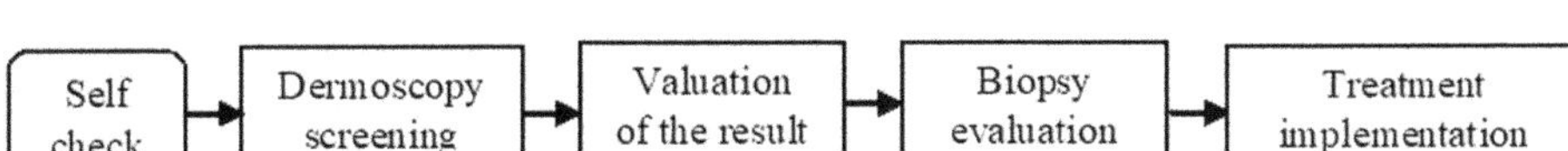

FIGURE 3.10 Clinical level detection of skin melanoma

3.2.4 Examination of Lungs

Lung is one of the fundamental interior organs in charge to provide the oxygen to the human physiology. The reason of the respiratory arrangement is to force oxygen from the atmosphere and shift it into the bloodstream, and to release carbon dioxide from the bloodstream into the atmosphere, in an exercise of gas exchange. Humans have two lungs, a right and left lung and are situated within the thoracic cavity of the chest. The right lung is bigger than the left, which shares space in the chest with the heart. The tissue of the lungs can be contaminated due to a number of respiratory diseases, including pneumonia and lung cancer. Recently emerged COVID-19 also infects the lungs with a substantial rate and causes medium/heavy pneumonia. The unprocessed lung disease will distress the respiratory system and disturbs the gas exchange among the bloodstream and atmosphere (Rajinikanth et al., 2020b; 2020c; Kadry et al., 2020; Ahuja et al., 2020).

A radiograph (chest X-ray or chest film) is generally used to recognize numerous conditions relating the chest wall, lungs, heart, and great vessels. The previous work verifies that, pneumonia and congestive heart fault are usually diagnosed by chest X-ray. Usually, the chest X-ray is appropriate to record and assess the normal/abnormal situation of the chest and it provides a fine screening output for further diagnosis. This sub-section depicts the chest X-ray of the pneumonia and tuberculosis cases collected from the benchmark datasets (Rajpurkar et al., 2018).

3.2.4.1 Pneumonia Diagnosis

Pneumonia arises due to the disease in the respiratory territory due to the microorganisms, such as bacteria, virus and fungi. The pneumonia causes a variety of defects in respiratory arrangement and prevents the oxygen switch to the bloodstream. The unprocessed pneumonia is extremely acute for the children (age <5 years) and elderly people (>65 years). In order to supply suitable treatment for the affected people, it is necessary to diagnose the lung disease rate in the lung. Due to its clinical importance, an extensive amount of semi-automated and automated disease finding schemes are proposed and executed to identify various lung irregularities with the chest X-ray [4].

Figure 3.11 depicts the chest X-ray obtained from the pneumonia database available at (Irvin et al., 2019). Figure 3.11 (a) and (b) depicts the healthy and pneumonia cases respectively. This radiograph slides are then scrutinized with suitable technique to measure the fault.

3.2.4.2 Tuberculosis Diagnosis

Tuberculosis (TB) is one of the sensitive lung sickness caused due to a bacteria named mycobacterium tuberculosis. The TB usually infects the lung and creates extremely acute respiratory disorder and in some particular cases, the TB disease can be seen in other body organs too. The assessment of the TB is usually done using; (i) Imaging technique, (ii) Endoscopy supported diagnosis and (iii) Needle biopsy. The typical chest radiograph of the TB can be found in Figure 3.11 (c).

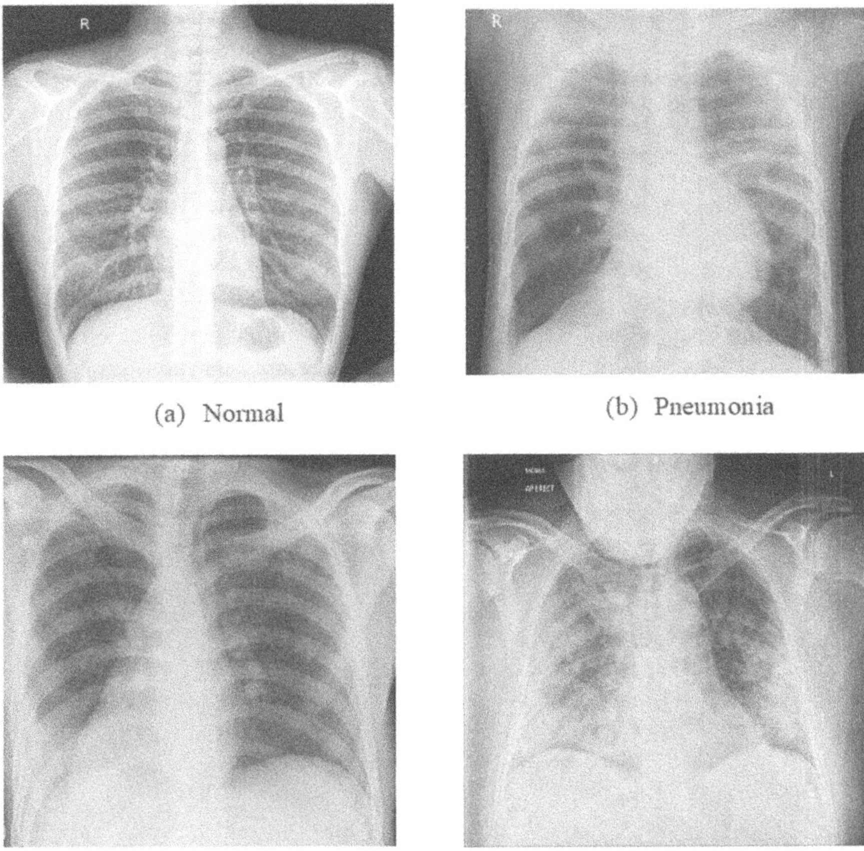

(a) Normal (b) Pneumonia

(c) Tuberculosis (d) COVID-19

FIGURE 3.11 Chest radiograph (X-ray) of healthy and abnormal lung sections

3.2.4.3 COVID-19 Infection

Recently emerged infectious Coronavirus Disease (COVID-19) emerged as one of the widespread global hazard and infected a large human society worldwide and due to its speedy stretch. The COVID-19 usually affects the human's respiratory tract and causes the sensitive pneumonia. The symptoms of the COVID-19 depend on patient's immunity and the frequent symptoms vary from dry cough to complexity in breathing.

The Disease Screening (DS) for COVID-19 includes two stages; (i) Reverse transcription-polymerase Chain Reaction (RT-PCR) test, and (ii) Image assisted diagnosis to substantiate the disease. RT-PCR is a laboratory level detection process performed using the samples collected from the infected patient. When the outcome by the RT-PCR is positive, then the doctor will advise an image assisted analysis to verify the disease and its harshness stage. During the image assisted analysis, the infection in lung will be recorded by means of Computed-Tomography (CT) scan images and/or chest radiographs (Chest X-Ray). The recorded images are then examined by an experienced doctor and based on his observation, the treatment planning and execution is performed. Figure 3.11 (d) depicts the chest X-ray of the infected patient. The infection severity can be examined by a radiologist followed by a doctor and based on this result; an appropriate treatment is designed and executed to treat the patient.

Computed Tomography (CT) scan is one of the extensively accepted imaging methods in hospitals to examine a range of organs, including the lungs. The chief benefit of CT is it offers a reconstructed 3D image which can be examined either in 3D or 2D form (Figure 3.12). The appraisal of the CT helps to recognize the disease precisely compared to the chest X-ray. From the literature, it can be noted that, the CT scan slices of axial, coronal and sagittal views are used for the assessment and the choice of a particular orientation depends on the doctor.

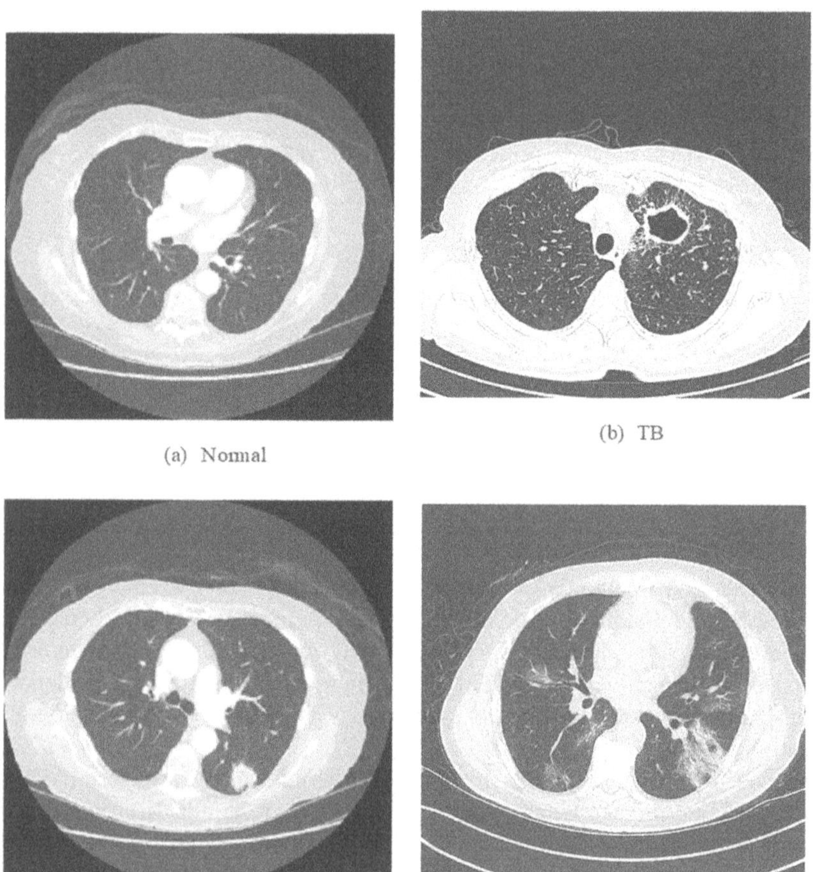

(a) Nomal

(b) TB

(c) Cancer

(d) COVID-19

FIGURE 3.12 Lung CT scan images of healthy and disease cases

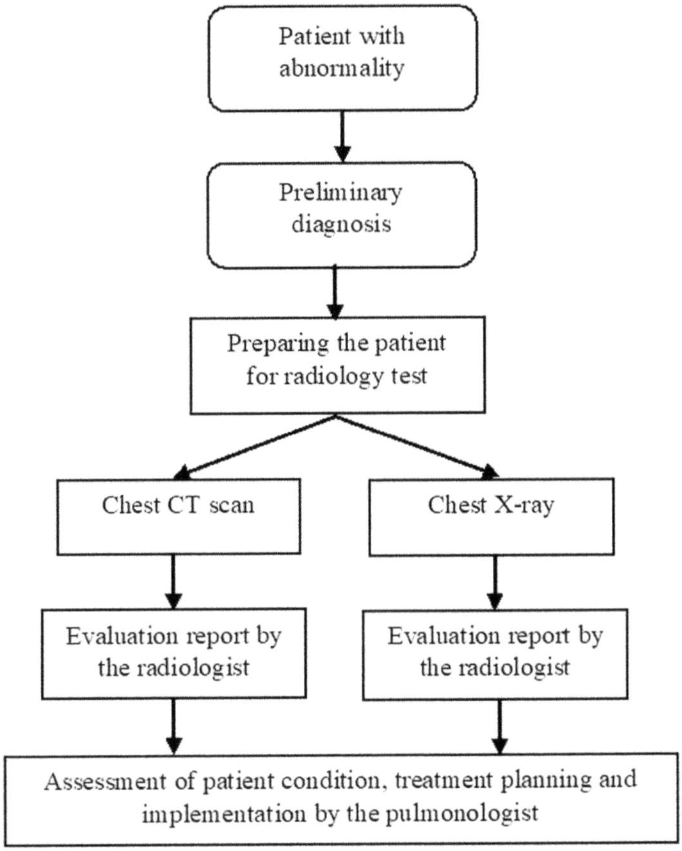

FIGURE 3.13 Clinical stage screening of the lung defects

The malformation in lung will severely affects the respiratory arrangement and agitates the air exchange. The shortage of oxygen in bloodstream will decrease the usual activities of other parts and the action of the cells will be troubled. If this problem continues, the physiology will be affected badly and it will lead to organ failure and death.

The defect in lungs is usually diagnosed with the CT scan or the chest X-ray, since it is covered with a complex bone section called the ribs, which holds and protects the lungs as well as the heart. The clinical level imaging system followed in radiology to record the activity and condition of the lungs is depicted in Figure 3.13. By employing this procedure, the 2D or 3D version of the image is recorded and then assessed by a doctor or a computer algorithm, to detect the abnormality with better accuracy.

3.2.5 Examination of Brain

In human physiology, brain is the chief organ, which is in charge to evaluate the entire physiological signal coming from other sensory sections and take the essential managing actions. This process is poorly affected, if any illness or disease arises in brain and the unnoticed and unprocessed brain sickness may lead to a variety of troubles including the death. The standard state of the brain may be affected due to a variety of causes, such as birth imperfection, head wound due to accident and the cell growth in heart of brain segment. Due to the diverse defensive schemes and the convenience of the contemporary caring conditions, the child with the birth defects is significantly condensed.

Newly, a substantial amount of alertness programs and the anticipatory measures are taken to protect the brain from malformation. But, due to an assortment of inescapable grounds, such as current life style, food behaviour, genetics and age; most of the humans are distress due to a variety of brain defects. If the brain defect is detected in its premature stage, then achievable measures can be executed to control the illness. The brain normally has a large amount of soft tissues along with the connected signal transceivers and hence, the biopsy is not suggested to identify these abnormalities (Rajinikanth et al., 2017; 2020d; Pugalenthi et al., 2019).

The defect in the brain will direct to a variety of irregularities in the arrangement, such as the difficulty in regular behaviours, speech, walking pattern and quick decision making. The unprocessed brain defect may cause the momentary and permanent disability in humans and some brain abnormalities will cause death.

The troubles in the brain are typically assed with the brain signals and the brain images and the medical level assessment of the signal/image assisted brain condition monitoring is very important. Figure 3.14 depicts the predictable procedures to be followed to verify the activity of the brain using a selected practice. The image assisted technique, such as MRI and CT is widely preferred due to its straightforwardness in the analysis of the brain state and these images are examined by a radiologist and a doctor and the combined decision by the radiologist and the doctor is then considered to plan for the treatment to cure the abnormality. The option of a preferred (image/signal) process depends chiefly on the doctor.

The assessment of the brain illness with imaging practice is quite straightforward due to its improved visibility and varied modality during the recording. This subsection presents the information on the appraisal of the brain tumor and stroke using the MRI and Computed-Tomography (CT) recorded images.

3.2.5.1 CT Scan

Computed Tomography (CT) imaging is extensively considered to record the brain images for the additional evaluation. Figure 3.15 (a) depicts the CT scan slices with brain tumor collected from the Radiopaedia database. Like the MRI, the CT scan also one of the radiology assisted imaging procedure widely considered by the radiologist and doctors to measure the malformation in brain with improved accuracy.

3.2.5.2 MRI

The evaluation of the brain irregularity is very commonly executed by means of the MRI due to its varied modalities, such as Flair, T1, T1C, T2 and the DW. Figure 3.15 (b) and (c) depicts the T2 modality images of the brain tumour images, such as Glioblastoma Multiforme (GBM) and the Low Grade Glioma (LGG) existing

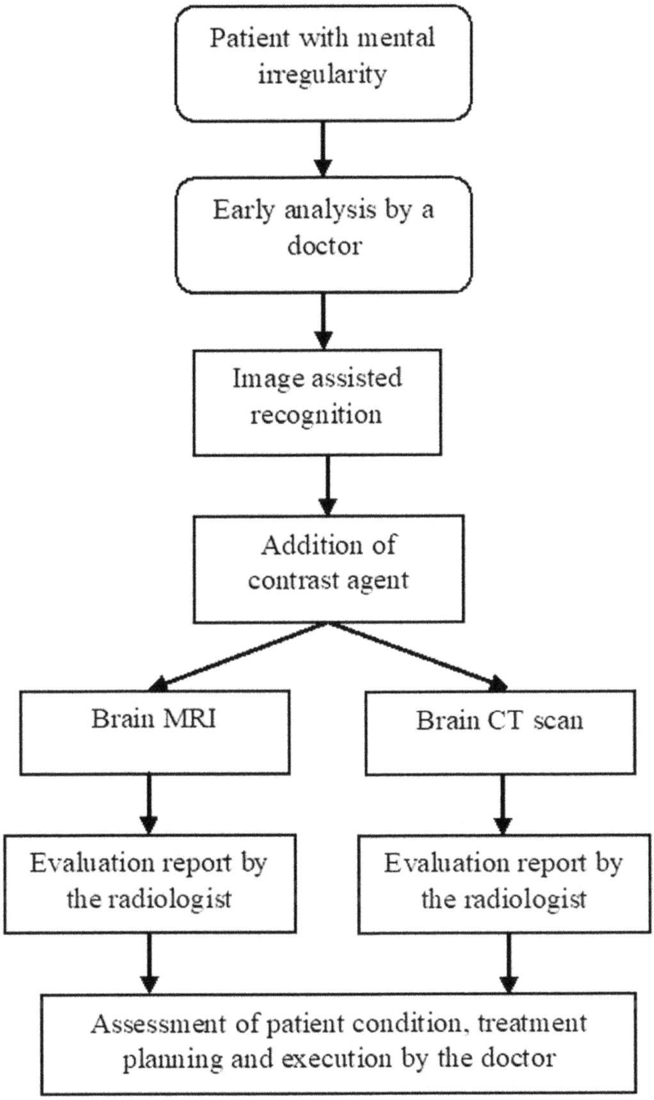

FIGURE 3.14 Clinical level diagnosis of the brain abnormality with signal/image based techniques

in the TCIA database (Pedano, et al., 2016). This dataset offers the clinical grade MRI images collected from the volunteers using a prescribed protocol.

During the recording of the MRI, a contrast agent called the Gadolinium is injected into the patient, which helps to record the abnormal section with better contrast compared to other brain sections. In Figure 3.15 (d), the flair modality images with ischemic stroke section is presented. All these abnormalities are evaluated using a suitable image assisted techniques.

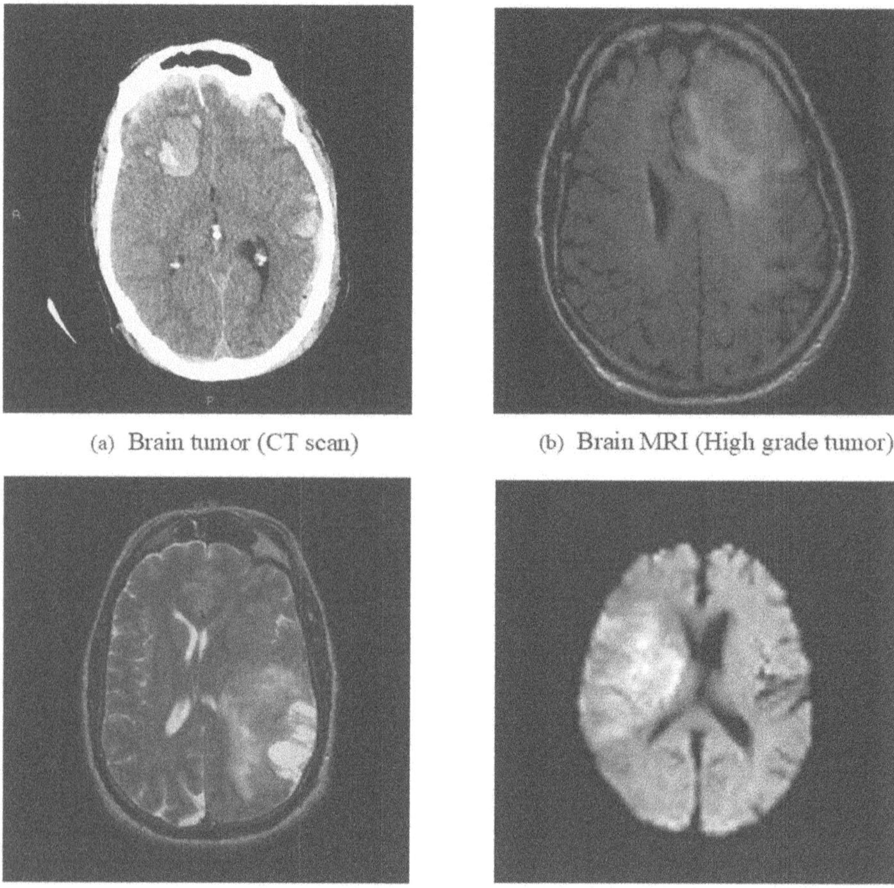

(a) Brain tumor (CT scan)

(b) Brain MRI (High grade tumor)

(c) Brain MRI (Low grade tumor)

(d) Brain MRI (Ischemic stroke)

FIGURE 3.15 Sample test images of the brain section with abnormalities

3.2.6 Examination of Breast

Breast cancer is one of the defects in women and affects a huge population group each year. Accessibility of the current medical potential can help the women society to understand the asymmetrical cell growth in the breast part through the screening procedure. When the nature of breast irregularity is documented, it is possible to present suitable treatment to cure the disease. Breast cancer usually originates in breast cells and it forms in either the lobules or the ducts of the breast. The preliminary level of the breast cancer can be identified with the help of the irregularity called the Ductal Carcinoma In Situ (DCIS); which caused due to the occurrence of irregular cells inside a milk duct of the breast. DCIS is can be accounted as the initial form of the breast cancer. The clinical stage detection of the DCIS and the breast cancer is usually executed with the widespread imaging modalities, such as

Magnetic Resonance Imaging (MRI), mammogram, ultrasound imaging and the thermal imaging.

The mainstream of breast cancers commence in the breast tissue that are made up of glands for milk formation, known as lobules, and ducts that join the lobules to the nipple. Primarily the breast tumour is due to the uneven lump in the breast tissue called a tumour. Mammogram and MRI are the extensive radiology practices used to observe the grown tumours. These methods rarely may fail to notice the breast disease, when the cancer is in premature stage. Hence, in recent years, thermal imaging and sonography are extensively adapted to verify and analyse the breast tumour due to its risk-free as well as contactless nature.

3.2.6.1 Mammogram

Mammogram is one of the widely used techniques to verify the breast division. During this practice, a specifically designed X-ray is used to record the breast segment with the help of a traditional film based or the digital technique. Due to the accessibility of the modern X-ray systems, digital mammogram recording is widely executed to record the breast abnormality. The recorded mammogram is then appraised by the expert to notice the irregularity.

FIGURE 3.16 (a) presents the sample test image of the mini-MIAS database. This is one of the extensively accepted mammogram dataset to assess the breast abnormality. This dataset consists of a class of mammogram slices of dimension 1024x1024x1 pixels and during the assessment, it can be resized to a necessary dimension to reduce the calculation difficulty of the image assessment system employed to identify the breast abnormality.

3.2.6.2 Breast MRI

Figure 3.16 (b) show the sample breast MRI slices of the axial view extracted from a three-dimensional (3D) breast MRI existing at the Reference Image Database to Evaluate Therapy Response (RIDER) of The Cancer Imaging Archive (TCIA) dataset (Clark et al., 2013; Meyer et al., 2015). The RIDER-TCIA is one of the well accepted benchmark database widely adopted by the researchers to test the developed computerized tool. The assessment of the 3D breast MRI is computationally complex and hence 3D to 2D conversion is essential to evaluate the breast sections using a simplified computerized tool. The assessment of the 2D MRI can help to identify the tumour with improved accuracy. Another advantage of the MRI is, it can help to trace the breast division with various modalities and the recorded breast section can be effectively diagnosed to identify the infection level and the orientation of the cancer in the breast section.

3.2.6.3 Thermal Imaging

Thermal imaging is a current imaging practice, in which the infrared radiation (IR) is recorded by means of a selected method to construct the image of the breast section to be examined. Digital Infrared Thermal Imaging (DITI) is the type of thermography extensively used to record the abnormal breast section for the further evaluation. The level of the IR wave coming-out from the body organ mostly depends on its situation and the thermal camera can be used to confine the radiation

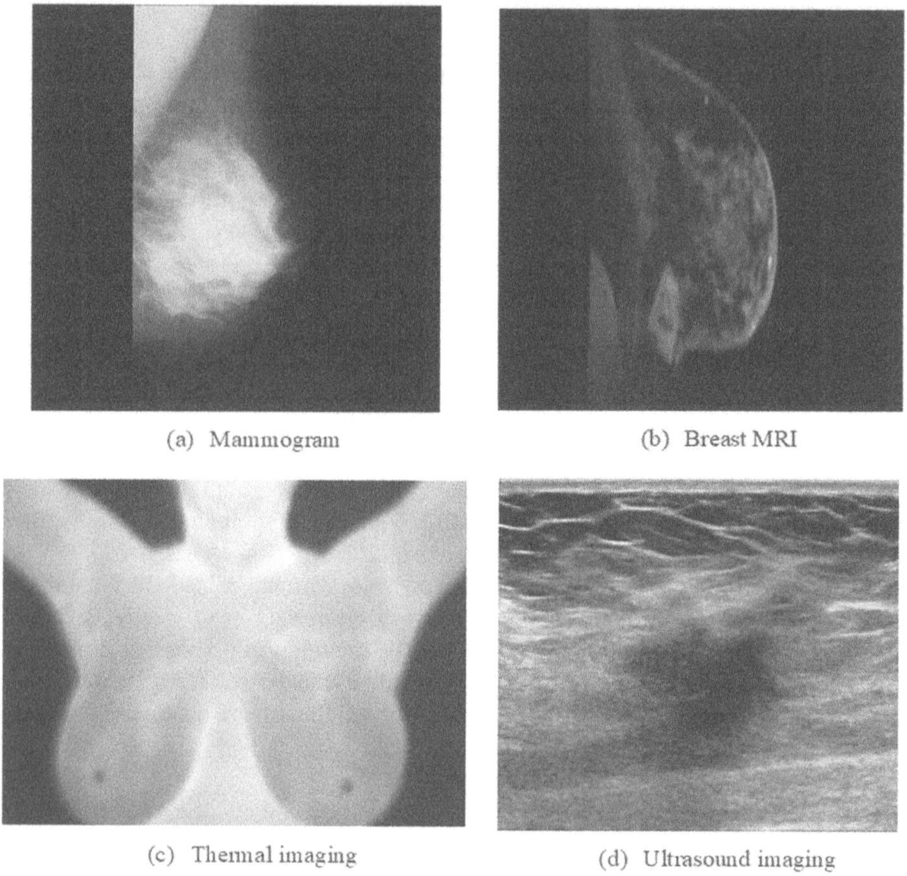

FIGURE 3.16 Various modalities to record the breast abnormality to detect the defects

and exchange it into image patterns using a dedicated software unit. The recorded thermal image will have a varied image pattern based on the level of the OR wave and by simply analysing its pattern, it is possible to detect the abnormality in the image. Figure 3.16 (c) presents the thermal images recorded using a chosen imaging modality. The earlier works on the breast thermogram analysis of the DCIS and the cancer can be found in (Fernandes et al., 2019; Raja et al., 2017; Silva et al., 2014; Rajinikanth et al., 2018).

3.2.6.4 Ultrasound Imaging

Over the two decades, the ultrasound imaging events are used in medical field to record the information and the activity of internal organs, tissues and the blood flow. This procedure uses high-frequency sound waves (sonography) to trace the necessary image [51]. Compared to former imaging modalities, it is proved to be very safe and will not cause any tissue level as well as the organ level damage. Recently, this imaging technique is widely adopted to screen a range of diseases including the breast abnormality. The ultrasound image of a breast section is depicted in Figure 3.16 (d).

As said earlier, the breast cancer arises in women due to different reasons, including ageing. When a woman is distress with a developed breast cancer; then the stage and the severity of the illness can be diagnosed with the help of a clinical biopsy, which helps to inspect the breast tissues and cells. Further, the image assisted technique with modalities, such as MRI, ultrasound, mammogram and thermal imaging is also used to inspect the breast irregularity with improved detection accuracy. These imaging techniques are non-invasive procedures and help to diagnose the disease with a visual examination by a doctor or with the help of a chosen computer algorithms. The detailed imaging procedure for the breast cancer detection is depicted in Figure 3.17.

3.3 CHOICE OF IMAGING MODALITY

In most of the diagnosis cases, the disease in a chosen body organ is recorded with preferred modalities for the further assessment. The choice of a particular imaging modality depends on the nature of the disease and its diagnosis level

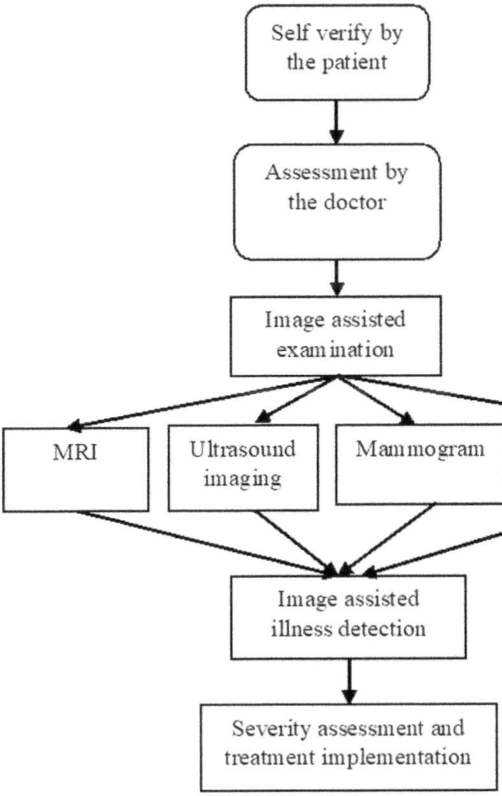

FIGURE 3.17 Clinical level breast cancer detection exercise

(organ/tissue level), health condition of the patient and the expertise of the doctor. Further, the imaging time and the cost also play a major role in some cases. If the patient condition is very severe, the rededication-based approaches may be avoided or a low radiation technique can be suggested to record the image with a compromised quality.

Let us consider the breast abnormality for the discussion. As presented in Figure 3.16, the breast abnormality can be assessed with a range of imaging techniques, such as mammogram, MRI, thermal imaging and ultrasound and the choice of the particular technique can be chosen as per the expertise of the doctor and the patient condition. The mammogram and the MRI are the radiological techniques commonly employed to record and analyse the abnormality in the breast section.

During the mammogram assisted detection; women's age and the breast density plays a major role, and in some cases the mammogram based detection will frequently offer false results, when it is executed on the women with lesser age. If the MRI is considered, the choice of the modalities, such as flair, T1, T1C, T2 and DW is quite difficult and it also needs expert's advice. Further, a contrast agent is to be injected into the human body to enhance the visibility of the infected breast section. The thermal imaging approaches are recent techniques, in which the IR radiation coming from the body is converted into RGB scaled pictures using a specialized camera and associated software. Due to its simplicity and adaptability, this technique is gaining the popularity in recent years. The ultrasound imaging is also one of the simple and widely preferred due to its merit. Every imaging technique has its own merit and demerits and the choice varies person to person based on the suggestion by the doctor.

The main motive of the imaging technique is to detect the abnormality in the organ and also detecting the disease and its severity with better diagnosing accuracy. The imaging procedure which supports the better detection with lesser effort is commonly recommended.

3.4 TRADITIONAL EXAMINATION

The commonly followed disease evaluation procedures are known as the common/traditional techniques. In this procedure, when a patient approaches the doctor with disease symptoms, the doctor will execute a sequence of examination procedures as per the general medical protocol. This procedures involves in; (i) personal verification, (ii) body temperature assessment, (iii) age, gender and weight assessment, (iv) assessment of the previous disease history, and (v) collecting and evaluation the blood samples to verify the blood level infection and the white-blood-cell count.

If the doctor gets any sign about the acute disease during this inspection, the doctor will suggest for the further check along with an image guided diagnosis to confirm the disease and its severity. After getting the test report from the scan centre and the imaging centre, the doctor will physically very the report with almost care and based on the finding, a treatment is suggested.

Normally, the outcome of the traditional examination procedure depends mainly on the assessment report by the doctor and the decision taken by the doctor is final. Even though this procedure offers better result, it is normally time consuming and the accuracy of the disease detection depends mainly on the doctor's experience. In most of the cases, a report needs to be verified and confirmed by more than one disease experts and this process is time consuming. Hence, in modern hospitals, along with the doctors, computerized algorithms are also used to analyse the disease condition and treatment suggestion. In most of the disease cases, the traditions examination methods are associated with modern technique to reduce the diagnosis time (Wang et al., 2004; Manikantan et al., 2012; Rajinikanth and Couceiro, 2015; Rajinikanth et al., 2013; 2019a).

3.5 COMPUTER ASSISTED ANALYSIS

The recent developments in the science and technology helped in improving the medical sector with better facilities. The rapid enhancement in computer and software domain also helped the medical sector by providing the support from patient screening to the treatment implementation. The advancement in computer domain also helped in the field-level and remote-level monitoring of the patient with better accuracy using the wearable sensors integrated using the Medical Internet of Things (MIoT) technique.

The role of the computers in disease diagnosis considerably reduced the burden of the doctors and helps to take the decision with reduced time. The rapid development in image and signal processing also helped to accomplish a better diagnosis with the help of the existing machine-learning and deep-learning techniques.

The Computer Assisted Disease Analysis (CADA) normally comprises a sequence of procedures to be executed by a computer algorithm and the final report of this scheme is verified and confirmed by the doctor. A normal computer assisted (machine-learning) scheme will include the following stages; (i) Pre-processing, (ii) Post-processing, (iii) Feature extraction and selection, (iv) Classifier implementation, and (v) Classification and disease detection.

In the literature, a number of CADA systems are proposed and implemented using a variety of procedures and the CADA developed for a particular disease case will not work for other cases. Further, the CADA are disease or image modality specific and will offer better diagnosis accuracy, when properly implemented. The usage of the CADA in modern hospitals is very common and this process considerably reduced the doctor's burden. Further, the usage of this procedure helps to take the decisions on treatment with reduced time and also this system considerably reduced the diagnostic cost.

3.6 PRE-PROCESSING AND POST-PROCESSING TECHNIQUES

The overall accuracy of the CADA scheme depends mainly on the image pre-processing and post-processing methods employed during the disease assessment. After recording the image of an organ using a selected imaging modality, it needs to be treated with a range of pre-processing steps to enhance the information. Even though a considerable amount of image pre-processing procedures are existing, this section outlines only the multi-level thresholding techniques, widely considered to enhance the disease infected section in medical images.

Image thresholding or multi-thresholding is extensively implemented in a variety of fields to pre-process the picture under study. A picture can be recognized as the plan of altered pixels with respect to the thresholds. In a digital picture, the allocation of the pixel plays a principal role and change or grouping of these pixels are very much preferred to enhance/change the information available in the image. In former days, the bi-level thresholding is selected to divide the raw image into two sections, such as Region of Interest (ROI) and the background. In this practice, the operator/computer algorithm is authorized to distinguish an Optimal-Threshold (OT) by means of a chosen function. Let, the specific picture has 256 thresholds (is ranging from 0 to 255) and from this, one threshold value is selected as the finest threshold as follows;

$$0 < OT < 255 \tag{3.1}$$

The chosen threshold will help to separate the picture into two sections; such as section 1 have the pixel distribution < *OT* and section 2 with pixel distribution > *OT*. This procedure divides the image into two-pixel groups and therefore, it is called as the bi-level thresholding.

If the plan is to separate the specified picture into more than two illustrations, then a multi-level thresholding is preferred. During this operation, the number of *OT* = number of threshold levels. For example, if a tri-level threshold is chosen for the study, it will separate the test image into three sections as depicted in Equation 3.2;

$$0 < OT_1 < OT_2 < 255 \tag{3.2}$$

In this case, the image is separated into three segments; such as section 1, (pixels between 0 *to* OT_1), section 2 (pixels between OT_1 *to* OT_2), and section 3 (pixels between OT_2 *to* *255*). In most of the applications, the information attained with the bi-level threshold is not appropriate and hence, a multi-thresholding is referred to pre-process greyscale/RGB images. The information on multi-level threshold can be found in the literature.

The post-processing of the image involves in extraction of the ROI using a chosen methodology. In this method, a chosen algorithm is considered to extract the pixel-group belongs to the ROI and after extracting the ROI, a specified analysis or a visual check is implemented to diagnose the disease. The commonly used segmentation procedures, such as watershed, active-contour, Chan-Vese, clustering technique and heuristic algorithm assisted segmentation falls under this category. From this section, it can be confirmed that the pre-processing enhances the ROI and the post-processing extract the ROI, which is essential during the detection and decision making.

3.7 SUMMARY

This part of the book presented information on a variety of diseases and the imaging modalities obtainable to detect the diseases in a variety of body organs. For each organ, a suitable imaging practice is to be executed to capture the picture of the organ with improved visibility under a controlled medical environment. Further, this section presented different procedures implemented to record and examine these images. From this section, it can be noted that, a number of imaging techniques are available for the disease screening process based on the organs and the choice of a particular procedure depends mainly on the expertise of the physician. The recorded images could be converted to digital and examined using a computer algorithm. This procedure aids the doctor to lessen the diagnostic burden. The outcome of the computerized practice as well as the observation by the doctor together would result in an efficient planning of the treatment, to control and cure the disease.

REFERENCES

Ahuja, S., Panigrahi, B. K., Dey, N., Rajinikanth, V., & Gandhi, T. K. (2020). Deep transfer learning-based automated detection of COVID-19 from lung CT scan slices. *Applied Intelligence.*

Bhandary, A., Prabhu, G. A., Rajinikanth, V., Thanaraj, K. P., Satapathy, S. C., Robbins, D. E., Shasky, C., Zhang, Y. D., Tavares, J. M. R. S., & Raja, N. S. M. (2020). Deep-learning framework to detect lung abnormality–A study with chest X-Ray and lung CT scan images. *Pattern Recognition Letters*, *129*, 271–278.

Chaki, J., & N Dey, N. (2020). Data tagging in medical images: A survey of the state-of-art. *Current Medical Imaging.*

Chavan, T., Sarma, G. R. K., & Rao, K. (2020, January). Enhanced single shot detector with image sharpening for detection of knee joint. In *Twelfth International Conference on Machine Vision (ICMV 2019)* (Vol. 11433, p. 114330C). International Society for Optics and Photonics.

Clark, K., Vendt, B., & Smith, K. et al. (2013). The Cancer Imaging Archive (TCIA): Maintaining and operating a public information repository, *Journal of Digital Imaging*, 26(*6*), 1045–1057.

Dey, N., Fuqian Shi, F., & Rajinikanth, V. (2019). Leukocyte Nuclei Segmentation Using Entropy Function and Chan-Vese Approach. *Information Technology and Intelligent Transportation Systems*, 314, 255–264.

Dey, N., Rajinikanth, V., Ashour, A. S., & Tavares, J. M. R. (2018). Social group optimization supported segmentation and evaluation of skin melanoma images. *Symmetry*, 10(*2*), 51.

Dougherty. (1994). *Digital Image Processing Methods*, CRC Press.

Fathima, S. N., Tamilselvi, R., & Beham, M. P. (2019). XSITRAY: A Database for the Detection of Osteoporosis Condition. *Biomedical and Pharmacology Journal*, 12(*1*), 267–271.

Fernandes, S. L., Rajinikanth, V., & Kadry, S. (2019). A hybrid framework to evaluate breast abnormality using infrared thermal images. *IEEE Consumer Electronics Magazine*, 8(5), 31–36.

Glaister, J. L. (2013). *Automatic segmentation of skin lesions from dermatological photographs* (Master's thesis, University of Waterloo).

http://peipa.essex.ac.uk/info/mias.html. (Accessed on: 15 March 2020).

http://visual.ic.uff.br/en/proeng/thiagoelias/# (Accessed on: 15 May 2020).

http://www.onlinemedicalimages.com/index.php/en/. (Accessed on: 15 May 2020).

https://uwaterloo.ca/vision-image-processing-lab/research-demos/skin-cancer-detection.

Irvin, J.et al., CheXpert: a large chest radiograph dataset with uncertainty labels and expert comparison. (2019). *arXiv:1901.07031* [cs.CV].

Kadry, S., Rajinikanth, V., Rho, S., Raja, N. S. M., Rao, V. S., & Thanaraj, K. P. (2020). Development of a Machine-Learning System to Classify Lung CT Scan Images into Normal/COVID-19 Class. *arXiv preprint arXiv:2004.13122.*

Kowsalya, N., Kalyani, A., Shree, T. V., Raja, N. S. M., & Rajinikanth, V. (2018). Skin-melanoma evaluation with Tsallis's thresholding and Chan-Vese approach. In *2018 IEEE International Conference on System, Computation, Automation and Networking (ICSCA)* (pp. 1–5). IEEE.

Manikantan, K., Arun, B. V., & Yaradonic, D. K. S. (2012). Optimal Multilevel Thresholds based on Tsallis Entropy Method using Golden Ratio Particle Swarm Optimization for Improved Image Segmentation, *Procedia Engineering*, 30, 364–371.

Marshall, D., Johnell, O., & Wedel, H. (1996). Meta-analysis of how well measures of bone mineral density predict occurrence of osteoporotic fractures. *Bmj*, 312(7041), 1254–1259.

McClung, M. R., Grauer, A., Boonen, S., Bolognese, M. A., Brown, J. P., Diez-Perez, A., & Katz, L.(2014). Romosozumab in postmenopausal women with low bone mineral density. *New England Journal of Medicine*, 370(5), 412–420.

Meyer, C. R., Chenevert, T. L., Galbán, C. J., Johnson, T. D., Hamstra, D. A., Rehemtulla, A., & Ross, B. D. (2015). Data From RIDER_Breast_MRI. The Cancer Imaging Archive.

Nair, M. V., Gnanaprakasam, C. N., Rakshana, R., Keerthana, N., & Rajinikanth, V. (2018, September). Investigation of breast melanoma using hybrid image-processing-tool. In *2018 International Conference on Recent Trends in Advance Computing (ICRTAC)* (pp. 174–179). IEEE.

Fathima, S. M., Tamilselvi, R., Parisa Beham, M., & Sabarinathan, D. (2020). Diagnosis of osteoporosis using modified U-net architecture with attention unit in DEXA and X-ray images. *Journal of X-Ray Science and Technology*, (Preprint), 1–21.

Pedano, N., Flanders, A. E., Scarpace, L., Mikkelsen, T., Eschbacher, J. M., Hermes, B., & Ostrom, Q. (2016). Radiology data from the cancer genome atlas low grade glioma [TCGA-LGG] collection. *Cancer Imaging Arch.*

Priya, E., & Srinivasan, S. (2015). Automated Identification of Tuberculosis Objects in Digital Images Using Neural Network and Neuro Fuzzy Inference Systems. *J Med Imag Health In*, 5, 506–512.

Priya, E., Srinivasan, S., & Ramakrishnan, S. (2014). Retrospective non-uniform illumination correction techniques in microscopic digital TB images. *Microsc Microanal*, 20(5), 1382–1391.

Pugalenthi, R., Rajakumar, M. P., Ramya, J., & Rajinikanth, V. (2019). Evaluation and classification of the brain tumor MRI using machine learning technique. *Control Eng. Appl. Inf*, 21, 12–21.

Raja, N. S. M., Rajinikanth, V., Fernandes, S. L., & Satapathy, S. C. (2017). Segmentation of breast thermal images using Kapur's entropy and hidden Markov random field. *Journal of Medical Imaging and Health Informatics*, 7(8), 1825–1829.

Rajinikanth, V., & Couceiro, M. S. (2015). RGB histogram based color image segmentation using firefly algorithm, *Procedia Computer Science*, *46*, 1449–1457.

Rajinikanth, V., Dey, N., Raj, A. N. J., Hassanien, A. E., Santosh, K. C., & Raja, N. (2020b). Harmony-search and Otsu based system for coronavirus disease (COVID-19) detection using lung CT scan images. *arXiv preprint arXiv:2004.03431.*

Rajinikanth, V., Kadry, S., Thanaraj, K. P., Kamalanand, K., & Seo, S. (2020c). Firefly-Algorithm Supported Scheme to Detect COVID-19 Lesion in Lung CT Scan Images using Shannon Entropy and Markov-Random-Field. *arXiv preprint arXiv:2004.09239.*

Rajinikanth, V., Lin, H., Panneerselvam, J., & Raja, N. S. M. (2020a). Examination of retinal anatomical structures—A study with spider monkey optimization algorithm. In *Applied Nature-Inspired Computing: algorithms and Case Studies* (pp. 177). Springer.

Rajinikanth, V., Madhavaraja, N., Satapathy, S. C., & Fernandes, S. L. (2017). Otsu's multi-thresholding and active contour snake model to segment dermoscopy images. *Journal of Medical Imaging and Health Informatics*, 7(8), 1837–1840.

Rajinikanth, V., Raj, A. N. J., Thanaraj, K. P., & Naik, G. R. (2020d). A customized VGG19 network with concatenation of deep and handcrafted features for brain tumor detection. *Applied Sciences*, 10(10), 3429.

Rajinikanth, V., Raja, N. S. M., & Arunmozhi, S. (2019a). ABCD rule implementation for the skin melanoma assessment–a study. In *2019 IEEE International Conference on System, Computation, Automation and Networking (ICSCAN)* (pp. 1–4). IEEE.

Rajinikanth, V., Raja, N. S. M., & Latha, K.(2014). Optimal multilevel image thresholding: an analysis with PSO and BFO algorithms. *Aust. J. Basic and Appl. Sci*, 8(9), 443–454.

Rajinikanth, V., Satapathy, S. C., Dey, N., Fernandes, S. L., & Manic, K. S. (2019). Skin melanoma assessment using Kapur's entropy and level set—a study with bat algorithm. In *Smart intelligent computing and applications* (pp. 193). Springer.

Rajinikanth, V., Satapathy, S. C., Fernandes, S. L., & Nachiappan, S. (2017). Entropy based segmentation of tumor from brain MR images—a study with teaching learning based optimization. *Pattern Recogn. Lett.* 94, 87–95.

Rajinikanth, V., Thanaraj, K. P., Satapathy, S. C., Fernandes, S. L., & Dey, N. (2019a). Shannon's entropy and watershed algorithm based technique to inspect ischemic stroke wound. *Smart Innovation, Systems and Technologies*, 105, 23–31.

Rajinikanth, V., et al. (2018). Thermogram assisted detection and analysis of ductal carcinoma in situ (DCIS). In: International Conference on Intelligent Computing, Instrumentation and Control Technologies (ICICICT) (pp. 1641–1646). IEEE.

Rajinikanth, V., Dey, N., Kavallieratou, E., & Lin, H. (2020) Firefly Algorithm-Based Kapur's Thresholding and Hough Transform to Extract Leukocyte Section from Hematological Images. In: Dey, N. (eds) Applications of firefly algorithm and its variants. *Springer Tracts in Nature-Inspired Computing*, 221–235. Springer.

Rajpurkar, P., Irvin, J., Ball, R. L., Zhu, K., Yang, B., Mehta, H., & Patel, B. N. (2018). Deep learning for chest radiograph diagnosis: A retrospective comparison of the CheXNeXt algorithm to practicing radiologists. *PLoS Medicine*, 15(11), e1002686.

Satapathy, S. C., Raja, N. S. M., Rajinikanth, V., Ashour, A. S., & Dey, N. (2018). Multi-level image thresholding using Otsu and chaotic bat algorithm. *Neural Computing and Applications*, 29(12), 1285–1307.

Shree, T. V., Revanth, K., Raja, N. S. M., & Rajinikanth, V. (2018). A hybrid image processing approach to examine abnormality in retinal optic disc. *Procedia Computer Science, 125*, 157–164.

Shriranjani, D., Tebby, S. G., Satapathy, S. C., Dey, N., & Rajinikanth, V. (2018). Kapur's entropy and active contour-based segmentation and analysis of retinal optic disc. In *Computational Signal Processing and Analysis* (pp. 287). Springer.

Silva, L. F. et al. (2014). A new database for breast research with infrared image, *J. Med. Imag. Health Inform*, 4(1), 92–100.

Sudhan, G. H. H., Aravind, R. G., Gowri, K., & Rajinikanth, V. (2017), January. Optic disc segmentation based on Otsu's thresholding and level set. In *2017 International Conference on Computer Communication and Informatics (ICCCI)* (pp. 1–5). IEEE.

Wang, Z., Bovik, A. C., Sheikh, H. R., & Simoncelli, E. P. (2004). Image quality assessment: from error measurement to structural similarity. *IEEE Trans Image Process*, 13(1), 1–14.

4 Entropy Techniques in Image Analysis

After obtaining the images using a suitable modality, it is necessary to implement the essential image processing procedure to enhance and extract the vital information from the images. In the literature, a number of image enhancement procedures are proposed and implemented separately for the greyscale and RGB scale pictures. The RGB image enhancement techniques will work on a class of greyscale images without further modifications. But, the enchantment methods of the greyscale picture may not work on RGB scale images and in most of the cases, a RGB to greyscale conversion is necessary during the execution. In recent years, most of the imaging procedures offers the RGB scale images and the RGB to greyscale conversion may decrease the vital information in the test image. Hence, to process the images without any negotiation, a number of image processing procedure are proposed separately for the greyscale and RGB scale pictures (Satapathy et al., 2018; Dey et al., 2020; Fernandes et al., 2019; Raja et al., 2017; Rajinikanth et al., 2017).

Bi-level and multi-level image thresholding is a proven image pre-processing technique widely adopted to enhance the essential information of the picture based on a chosen threshold value from the histogram assisted evaluation. The histogram is a scientific representation of the image and it can be constructed by keeping the thresholds in X-axis and pixel value in Y-axis (Balan et al., 2016; Monisha et al., 2019; Rajinikanth et al., 2020).

During the image enhancement based on multi-level thresholding procedure; the threshold values of the images are arbitrarily varied till the information in the image is enhanced to an accepted level. The enhanced information is then considered to evaluate the image under study. From the literature, it can be noted that the implementation of the multi-level thresholding applicable for the greyscale image is quite simple compared to the GB scale image, due to its histogram pattern. In the RGB scale, a separate histogram exists for the image pixels, such as R, G, and B. The earlier research works related to the multi-level thresholding confirms that; there exist a number of thresholding procedures to process the image and these procedures are grouped as; (i) Entropy based method and (ii) Non-entropy-based method. According to the need and the expertise of the operator, a chosen technique is considered to enhance the image under examination. The earlier research works confirms that, the entropy assisted technique will offer a better result compared to the non-entropy-based approaches.

The main role of the entropy technique is to enhance the ROI when an appropriate image pre-processing is executed. Commonly, the multi-level thresholding procedures are executed to enhance the test image using an entropy and non-entropy-based methods and the literature confirms that the outcome attained with the entropy-based technique is superior compared to the alternative. This chapter of the book presents the commonly employed entropy assisted thresholding procedures with appropriate examples. The entropy-assisted threshold is executed separately for the greyscale and RGB scale medical pictures and the attained outcome is assessed using appropriate techniques.

4.1 EVALUATION OF MEDICAL IMAGES

In therapeutic field, images recorded using a chosen modality with a preferred pixel level can be considered to express important information. In some situations, the information existing in the unprocessed images are hard to distinguish and hence a number of pre-processing and post-processing activities are proposed and performed by the researchers (Rajinikanth et al., 2018; Shree et al., 2018; Fernandes et al., 2019a). The implemented picture processing methods can assist to develop the state of the unprocessed picture by means of a selection of methodologies, such as edge-detection, noise-removal, contrast enrichment, and thresholding. Due to its status and practical importance, a selection of grey/RGB scale picture threshold selection methods are employed by the researchers to process the digital photographs recorded with varied modalities. A preferred thresholding practice will help to enhance the visibility of the illustration's part by grouping the related pixels according to the selected threshold value.

Conventional and soft-computing assisted multi-threshold is a recognized picture pre-processing scheme broadly adopted in the image processing literature to improve the visibility of the ROI in various test images. For the chosen test illustration of grey/RGB scale, the threshold value can be seen by plotting the histogram of the image. The histogram is a graphical demonstration of the pixel distribution (X-axis) of the illustration with respect to the threshold value (Y-axis). For simplicity, the frequently considered threshold value during the image examination task is chosen as $L = 256$. For each image, the threshold value is fixed and the pixel distribution will differ based on the size and information obtainable in the medical picture.

Let us chose a bone X-ray slice with a dimension of 512x512x1 pixels and the histogram of the picture symbolize the allocation of the image pixels with respect to the threshold. For this picture, the threshold level is achieved by employing the bi-level and multi-level threshold selection process and the results are clearly presented in Figure 4.1. In this image, Figure 4.1 (a) to (c) depicts the sample test image, histogram and the bi-level thresholded image respectively. From Figure 4.1 (c), it can be confirmed that, the thresholding procedure will improve the visibility of the image section even though it is associated with the noise. Other related information regarding the medical image thresholding can be found in the earlier research articles (Manikandan et al., 2014; Li et al., 2015; Feng et al., 2017).

Image thresholding procedure helps to enhance the pixel information of the digital image, which then can be predicted and analysed for additional evaluation. In medical field, thresholding procedure will divide the digital picture into background, normal section and section with the disease (ROI). Finally, the part with the disease can be extracted with a selected segmentation practice and examined further. The outcome of the Figure 4.1 confirms that, the proposed procedure works well on the images with/without noise and enhanced the ROI considerably.

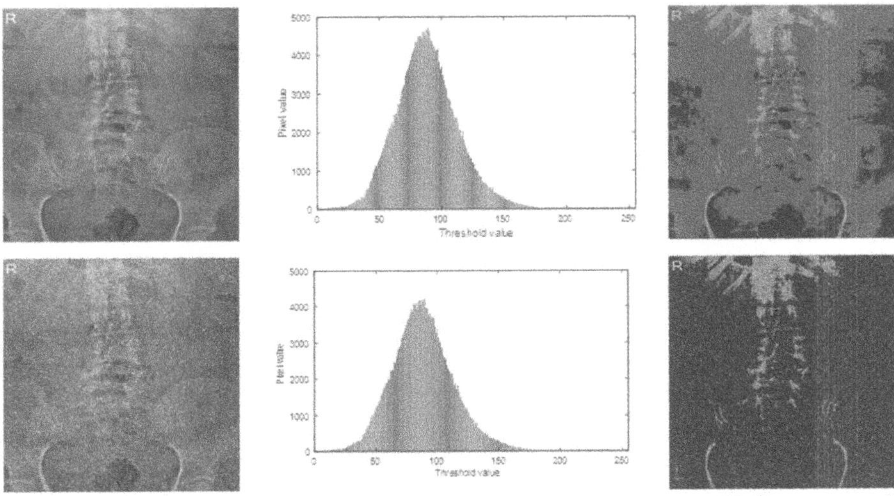

(a) Test image (b) Gray histogram (c) Pre-processed image

FIGURE 4.1 Thresholding result attained for image with and without the noise

4.2 GREY AND RGB SCALE IMAGES

The plan of the picture thresholding is to identify the finest/optimal threshold, which divide the image into a variety of classes based on the allocated threshold constraint. The threshold choice for the greyscale picture is straightforward compared to RGB, since, in greyscale case, implementation is easy but for RGB case, it is independently applied for the histograms of R, G and B respectively. According to the number of thresholds, it is classified as; (i) bi-level and (ii) multi-level thresholding and this practice is clearly presented in forthcoming part with suitable experimental results achieved with the MATLAB software.

For example, let us discuss the thresholding of bi-level class and it can be extended to the multi-level class with suitable modifications. Let, $Th = (T_0, T_1, ..., T_{L-1})$ demotes the number of thresholds obtainable in a selected digital picture of fixed aspect and every picture is to be assessed by considering its histogram created by the pixel distribution (Y-axis) and threshold distribution (X-axis). The thresholding process needs the recognition of a finest threshold value $Th = T_{OP}$, which supports the grouping of the picture pixels to improve the visibility of the ROI. The thresholding method can be implemented using (i) Bi-level approach (sorting into two groups) and (ii) Multi-level technique (sorting into multiple clusters).Based on the need, we can implement the bi-level as well as multi-level thresholding procedure on a chosen image.

Detection of a fitting practice to enhance the digital image is a reasonably demanding task and the appropriate image assessment techniques can be chosen based on the suggestion by the earlier works or by experience. In the literature, a number of threshold selection procedures are obtainable and the usually considered techniques are presented in Figure 4.2. Each method has its own qualities and in the literature,

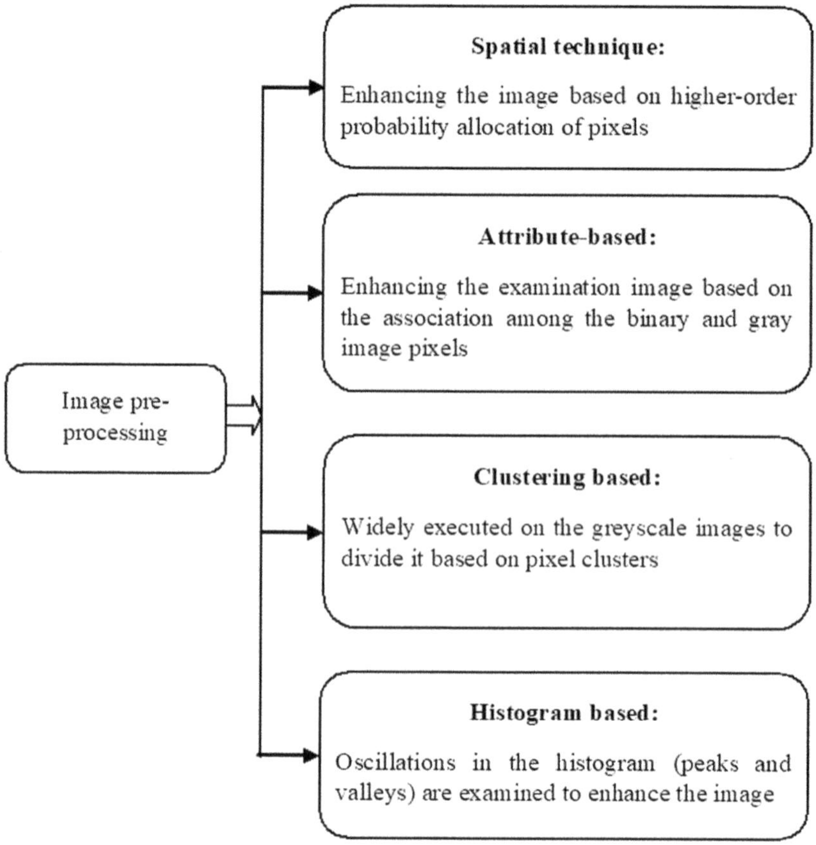

FIGURE 4.2 Common pre-processing procedures for image enhancement

histogram assisted threshold selection procedure is widely considered to enhance the greyscale/RGB scale picture compared to the alternatives. In the histogram supported thresholding procedure, the image histogram is examined with a selected technique, in which the threshold values are arbitrarily varied till the excellence of the processed image reaches to a confident stage. In this method, a selected objective value is taken as the guiding mechanism to justify the excellence of the picture based on a chosen image related measure. This measure is called the objective function.

In the histogram-based method, the difficulty of the thresholding augments due to the (i) size of the picture, (ii) pixel distribution, and (iii) multiple pixel class (ie, RGB). When the image dimension increase, the number of pixels in the image also will rise and which may increase the calculation time during the threshold choice, further the thresholding complexity also will increase with uneven pixel distribution (large peaks and valleys in histogram) and also the RGB class histogram.

Figures 4.3 and 4.4 depicts the chosen fundus test image of grey/RGB scale and the associated histograms. From this figure, it can be confirmed that, the histogram in RGB scale image is quite complex compared to the greyscale. Hence, during the

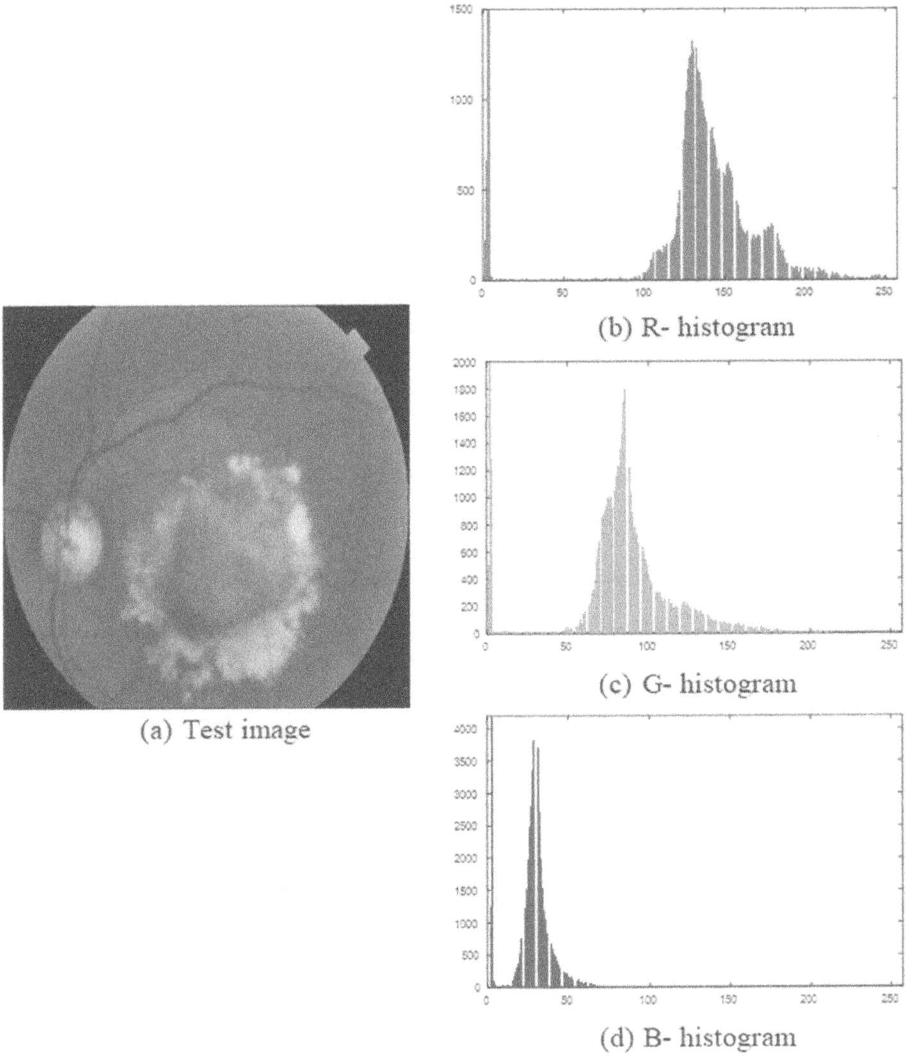

FIGURE 4.3 RGB scale retinal fundus image and its histogram

pre-processing task, separate thresholding methodology is to be executed for the RGB/grey images.

4.3 IMAGE PRE-PROCESSING

In recent years, a number of image pre-processing techniques are employed to enhance the medical grade pictures and this section the commonly used thresholding assisted image enhancement technique is discussed using the appropriate procedures with suitable examples.

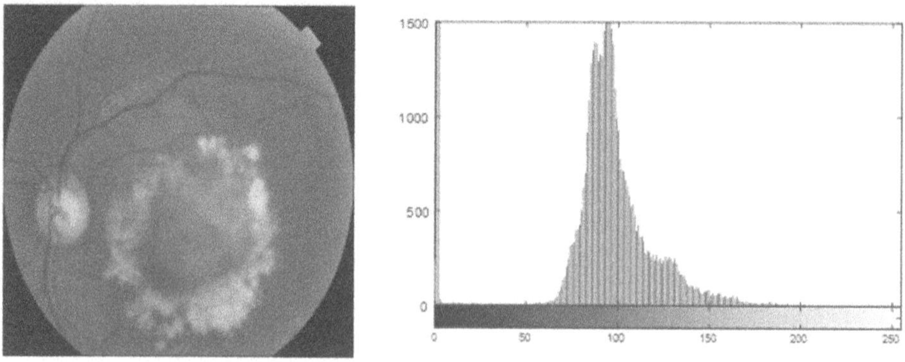

(a) Test image (b) Gray histogram

FIGURE 4.4 Greyscale retinal fundus image and its grey histogram

4.3.1 Entropy and Non-Entropy Based Pre-Processing

In the literature, the bi-level and multi-level thresholding is commonly executed to enhance the ROI of the test image. Based on the working mechanism, the threshold selection procedures are classified as the non-entropy based approach and the entropy based technique. The earlier research work confirms that, the entropy assisted ROI improvement procedures are preferable compared to the non-entropy assisted technique.

4.3.1.1 Otsu's Technique

Otsu's method was principally discussed in 1979 and it works based on between-class-variance idea and it recognizes the optimum threshold by maximizing the objective value (Otsu, 1979). The between-class-variance is the Otsu's non-parametric threshold choice theory, to be calculated by arbitrarily varying the picture threshold by means of a selected method. During this procedure, the selection of $Th = T_{OP}$ is necessary to exchange the raw picture into processed picture. This procedure works well on bi-level and multi-level threshold process for a class of greyscale and RGB scale images.

Let us chose a greyscale picture for the study. During the bi-level process; $Th = T_o, T_1$ are selected, which split the input image into two groups, such as J_0 and J_1 (background and ROI). The group J_0 contain the grey pixels of range 0 to T_o and class J_1 encloses the grey levels from T_1 to 255 (Rajinikanth and Couceiro, 2015;2015a). Otsu's technique works well on a class of greyscale and RGB scale images and helps to provide better outcome on a class of images remaining from the traditional benchmark images to the complex medical images (Acharya et al., 2019; Rajinikant et al., 2017; Rajinikanth and Satapathy, 2018; Dey et al., 2019; Roopini et al., 2018).

The mathematical expressed based on the probability sharing and its distribution for the grey pixels J_0 and J_1 can be designated as;

$$J_0 = \frac{P_0}{\eta_0(Th)} \cdots \frac{P_{T_0-1}}{\eta_0(Th)} \quad \text{and} \quad J_1 = \frac{P_{T_0}}{\eta_1(Th)} \cdots \frac{p_{255}}{\eta_1(Th)} \tag{4.1}$$

where $\eta_0(Th) = \sum_{i=0}^{Th-1} P_i$, $\eta_1(Th) = \sum_{i=Th}^{255} P_i$

The mean values; δ_0 and δ_1 for J_0 and J_1 can be represented by;

$$\delta_0 = \sum_{i=0}^{Th-1} \frac{iP_i}{\eta_0(Th)} \quad \text{and} \quad \delta_1 = \sum_{i=Th}^{255} \frac{iP_i}{\eta 1(Th)} \tag{4.2}$$

The Mean intensity (δ_{Th}) of the complete picture can be symbolized as:

$$\delta_{Th} = \eta_0\delta_0 + \eta_1\delta_1 \quad \text{and} \quad \eta_0 + \eta_1 = 1$$

The objective value for the bi-level thresholding is:

$$Otsu_{\max} = J(Th) = \vartheta_0 + \vartheta_1 \tag{4.3}$$

where $\vartheta_0 = \eta_0\ (\delta_0 - \delta_{Th})^2$ & $\vartheta_1 = \eta_1\ (\delta_1 - \delta_{Th})^2$

This method can be modified in the direction of a multi-level threshold by including various '*Th*' values.

Figure 4.5 presents the thresholding outcome attained using the Otsu's function. This technique is separately executed on the chosen greyscale and RGB scale image and the attained images are recorded. The optimal threshold selection is a quite time consuming task and hence, in the proposed work, social group optimization (SGO) is employed and the implementation of the SGO in multi-level thresholding can be found in (Satapathy and Naik, 2016; Dey et al., 2018; Naik et al., 2018). SGO has been formed by replicating the presentation and information conveying followed during human grouping for decision making. The SGO includes two chief functions, namely the (i) improving stage, and the (ii) acquiring stage.

The arithmetical model for the SGO is as follows:

Let us consider S_i as the initial information of people in an assembly and $i = 1, 2, 3, \ldots, H$, with H as the amount of people in the grouping. If the optimization task needs a D-dimensional exploration space, then the knowledge term can be expressed as $S_i = (S_{i1}, S_{i2}, S_{i3}, \ldots, S_{id})$. For any task, the fitness value can be defined as f_j, with $j = 1, 2, \ldots, H$. Thus, for the maximization problem, the fitness value can be written as:

$$Gbest_j = max\ \{f(S_i) \quad for \quad i = 1, 2, \ldots, H\} \tag{4.4}$$

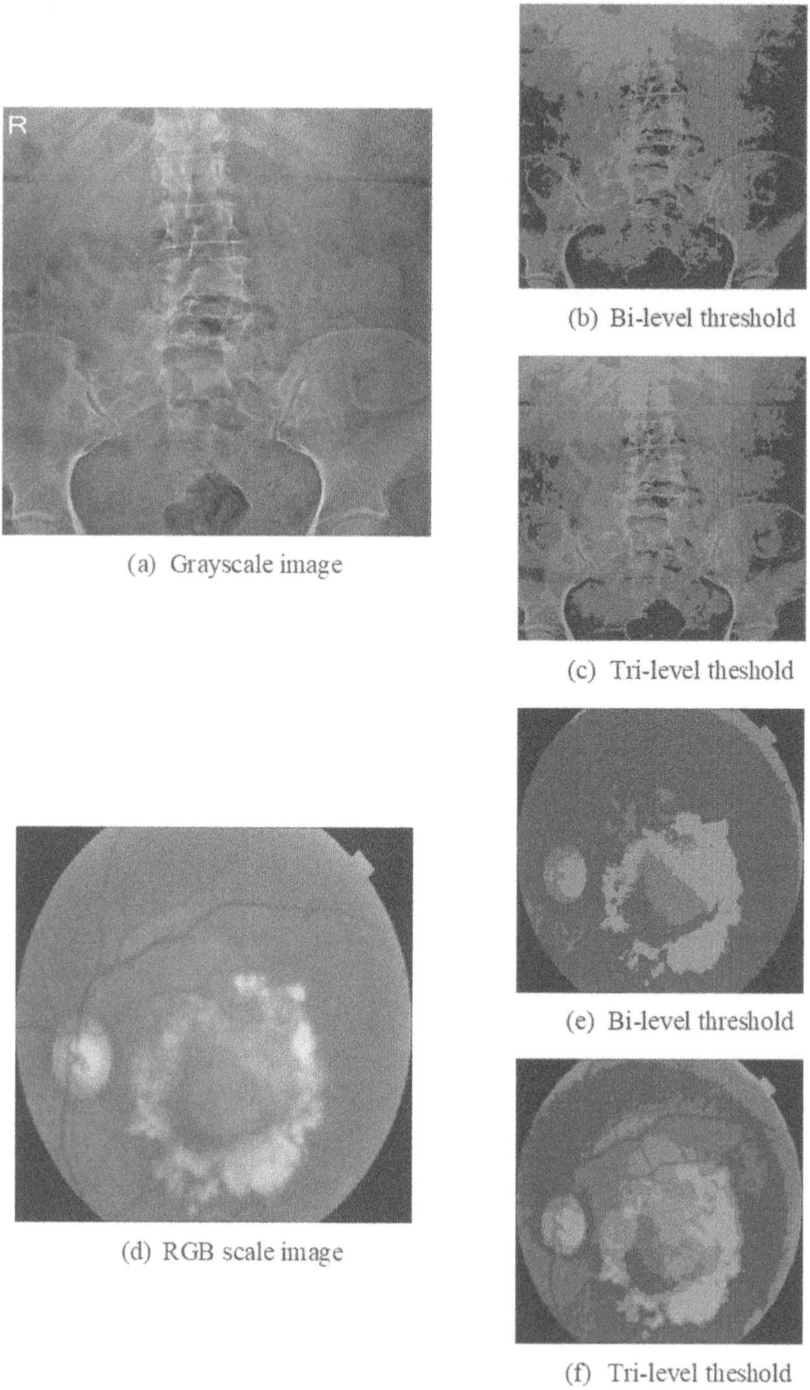

FIGURE 4.5 Otsu's based bi-level and tri-level thresholding

The steps of the normal SG algorithm can be illustrated as below;

Traditional SGO Algorithm

Start

Imagine five agents (*i =1,2,3,4,5*)

Allocate these agents to decide the $Gbest_j$ in a *D*-dimensional examination space

Arbitrarily allocate the whole agents in the collection all over the examination space during initialization practice

Calculate the fitness based on the task to besolved

Update the direction of agents with $Gbest_j = \max \{f(S_i)\}$

Start the improving phase to revise the information of additional agents in order to get the $Gbest_j$

Start the acquiring stage to proceed the information of agents by arbitrarily choosing the agents with finest fitness

Repeat the process till the whole agents travel towards the finest potential position in the *D*-dimensional investigation space

If all the agents contain roughly similar strength values ($Gbest_j$)

Then

conclude the search and exhibit the optimized outcome for the selected task

Else

Repeat the preceding steps

End

Stop

In order to modernize the location (information) of each individual in the cluster, the improving phase considers the following relation:

$$S_{new_{i,j}} = c * S_{old_{i,j}} + R * (Gbest_j - S_{old_{i,j}}) \tag{4.5}$$

where S_{new} = new information, S_{old} = old information, *Gbest* = global best information, *R* = arbitrary number [0,1], and *c* represents the self-introspection constraint [0,1] and its value is chosen as 0.2. Other information on SGO can be found in (Feng et al., 2016; Fang et al., 2018; Praveen et al., 2018).

Advantages: The Otsu's practice is one of the general and regularly used practices to enhance a range of images. This approach works well on greyscale images and helps to achieve improved values of picture excellence parameters compared to other related techniques.

Limitations: Even though, this method works on a variety of images, its performance is very less compared to the entropy-based techniques, when the abnormality of the image is the prime ROI. When the deformity is inspected, the entropy based method offers better result compared to the Otsu.

4.3.1.2 Kapur's Entropy

Kapur's technique has been principally proposed for thresholding the greyscale pictures by means of the histogram's entropy (Kapur et al., 1985; Kapur and Kesavan, 1992). This technique finds the finest threshold by maximizing the entropy.

Let for a chosen dimension of the greyscale image with L grey-levels (0 to $L-1$) with a total pixel value of Z. If $f(k)$ symbolizes the frequency of kth intensity-level; then the pixel distribution of the image will be:

$$Z = f(0) + f(1) + \cdots + f(L-1) \tag{4.6}$$

If the probability of kth intensity-level is given by:

$$p(k) = f(k) / Z \tag{4.7}$$

During the threshold selection, the pixels of image are separated into $T+1$ groups according to the assigned threshold value. After extrication the images as per the selected threshold, the entropy of each cluster is independently calculated and combined to get the final entropy as follows:

$$Bi-levelthreshold = f(t_1, t_2) = e_0 + e_1 \tag{4.8}$$

$$Multi-levelthreshold = f(t_1, t_2, ...t_L) = e_0 + e_1 + \cdots + e_{L-1} \tag{4.9}$$

$$\begin{aligned} e_0 &= -\sum_{k=0}^{k=t_1-1} \frac{p_k}{\sigma_0} \ln \frac{p_k}{\sigma_0}, \sigma_0 = \sum_{k=0}^{k=t_1-1} p_k \\ e_1 &= -\sum_{k=t_1-1}^{k=t_1-2} \frac{p_k}{\sigma_1} \ln \frac{p_k}{\sigma_1}, \sigma_1 = \sum_{k=t_1-1}^{k=t_1-2} p_k \\ e_{L-1} &= -\sum_{k=t_{L-1}}^{k=t_{L-2}} \frac{p_k}{\sigma_{L-1}} \ln \frac{p_k}{\sigma_{L-1}}, \sigma_{L-1} = \sum_{k=t_{L-1}}^{k=t_{L-2}} p_k \end{aligned} \tag{4.10}$$

where e = entropy, p = probability distribution, and σ = probability occurrence.

$$Kapur_{\max}(T) = \sum_{p=1}^{L-1} H_j^C \tag{4.11}$$

Other information on Kapur's function can be found in (Manic et al., 2016; Shriranjani et al., 2018).

SGO and Kapur's based thresholding is then executed on the medical grade images such as the bone X-ray and fundus retinal images and the related results are depicted in Figure 4.6. From Figure 4.6 (a) and (b), it can be observed that the proposed thresholding operation clearly enhances the ROI in the test images considerably in both the greyscale and RGB scale images. To confirm the superiority of the outcome, a comparative assessment between the original test image and the enhanced image is to be performed and based on the attained result; the superiority of the chosen thresholding procedure is confirmed.

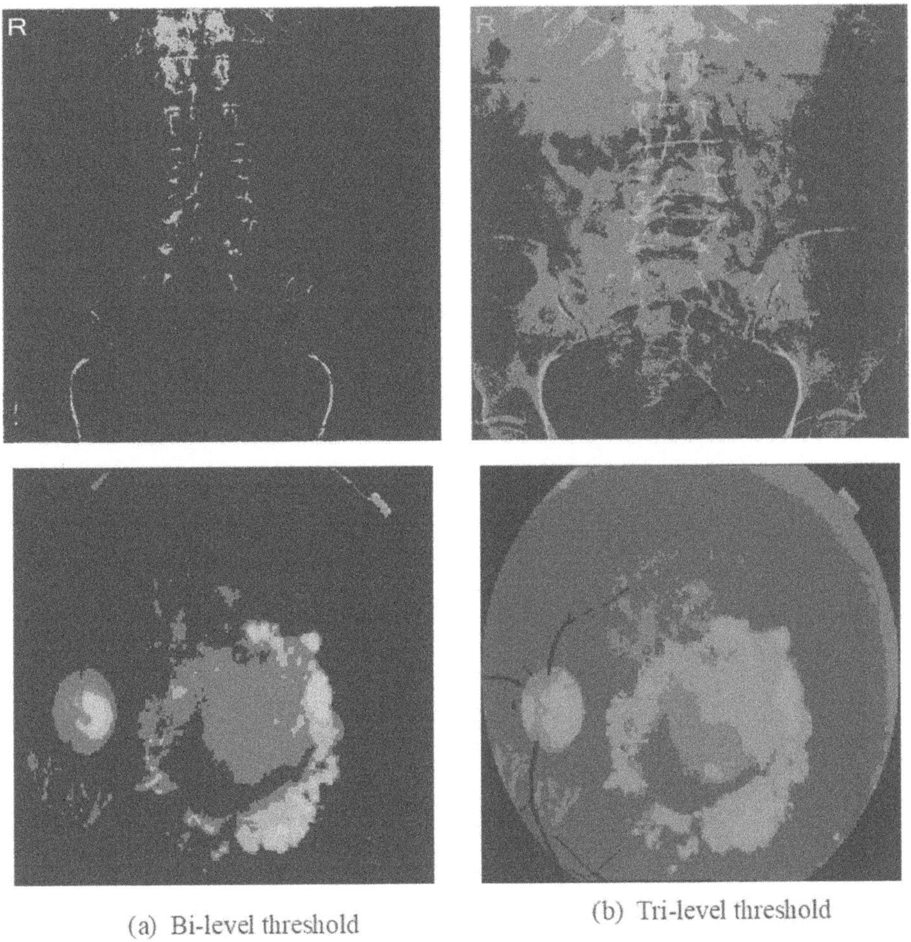

FIGURE 4.6 Kapur's based bi-level and tri-level thresholding outcome

Advantages: It is one of the extensively considered entropy and provides improved result on a class of greyscale and RGB images.

Limitations: The picture quality measures attained with this technique is poor compared to other methods.

4.3.1.3 Tsallis Entropy

Usually, entropy is associated with the computation of chaos in an arrangement. Shannon initially measured the entropy-based appraisal to calculate the hesitation concerning the series substances of the scheme (Plastino and Plastino, 1993). Shannon assured that, when a substantial structure is detached as two statistically free subsystems A_1 and A_2, then its entropy can be expressed as (Pugalenthi et al., 2019):

$$S_h(A_1 + A_2) = S_h(A_1) + S_h(A_2) \tag{4.12}$$

From above equation, a non-extensive entropy-based concept was introduced by Tsallis as shown below:

$$S_{hQ} = \frac{1 - \sum_{i=1}^{T} (P_i)^Q}{Q - 1} \tag{4.13}$$

where T = threshold and Q = entropic index. Eq. (4.12) will meet the Shannon's entropy when $Q \rightarrow 1$.

Other related information on Tsallis entropy can be found in earlier works (Lakshmi et al., 2016; Raja, et al., 2018).

Figure 4.7 presets the results attained using the SGO and Tsallis entropy-based thresholding for an assigned threshold values of $Th = 2$ (bi-level) and $Th = 3$ (tri-level).

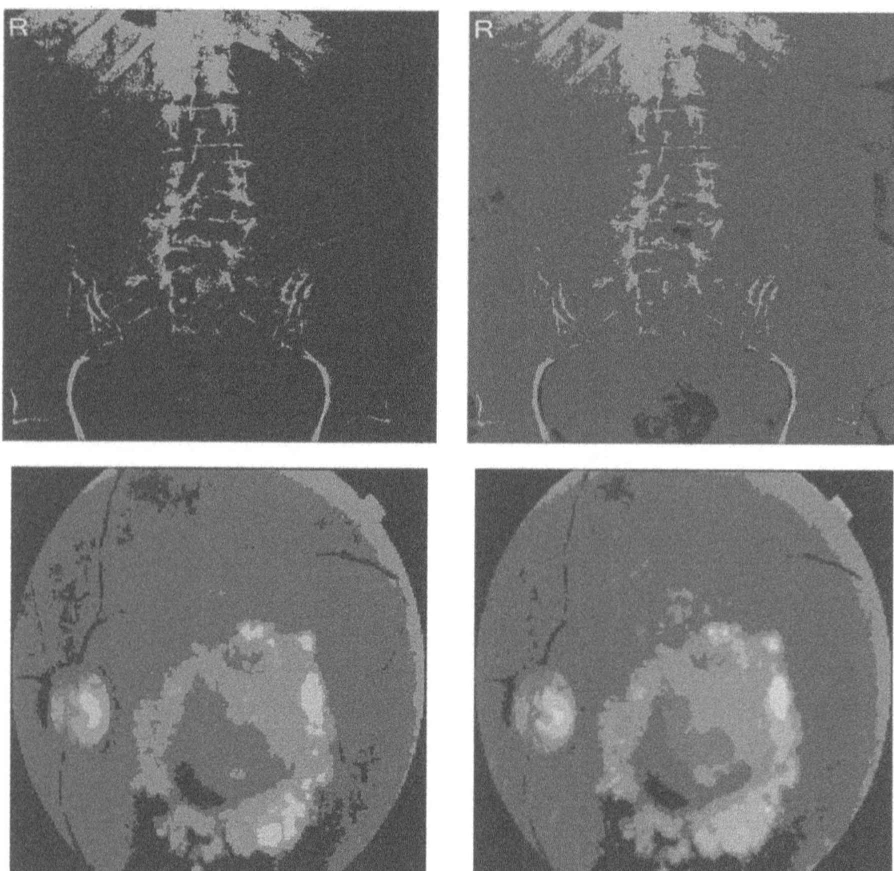

(a) Bi-level threshold (b) Tri-level threshold

FIGURE 4.7 Tsallis's entropy based bi-level and tri-level thresholding

The Tsallis scheme randomly varies the thresholds of the given image till the maximum value of the entropy is attained. When a maximized entropy is achieved by this operation, the optimization search stops and the results are displayed. The information (ROI) available in the thresholded image is then extracted using a chosen segmentation process and then it is assessed using a computer software. The other information regarding the SGO and Tsallis thresholding based medical image assessment can be accessed from the related earlier works (Raguram, et al., 2018).

Advantages: Entropy supported practice works fine on a class of images and particularly, it offers improved result during the picture irregularity assessment task.

Limitations: Compared to other methods, the picture quality measures achieved with the Tsallis function is very less and the grouping of the pixel achieved with this technique is poor compared to the Shannon's technique.

4.3.1.4 Shannon's Entropy

In the Shannon's Entropy (SE), let us decide a test-picture of dimension X*Y. The pixel organization in test-picture (x,y) is defined as F(x,y), for $x \in \{1,2,...,X\}$ & $y \in \{1,2,...,Y\}$. Let L is amount of grey-levels of the test-picture and the set of every grey values $\{0,1,2,..., L-1\}$ can be indicate D as O, in such a way that:

$$F(X,Y) \in O \quad \forall (x,y) \in Image \tag{4.14}$$

Then, the normalized histogram will be:

$$S = (T_0, T_1, ..., T_{L-1}). \tag{4.15}$$

For a bi-level thresholding case, Eqn. (4.15) becomes:

$$S(Th) = a_0(T_1) + a_1(T_2) \tag{4.16}$$

$$E(Th) = \max_{Th} \{S(Th)\} \tag{4.17}$$

where, $Th = \{T_1, T_2,..., T_L\}$ is the threshold value, $S = \{a_0, a_1,..., a_{L-1}\}$ is the normalized histogram, and $E(T)$ is the optimal threshold. For an RGB image case, the above technique is separately implemented for the R, G, and B threshold cases. Other information on the SE can be found in (Lin,1991; Wu et al., 2013).

Identification of the optimal threshold from a chosen image is a challenging task and this section presents the optimal threshold attained using the SGO and Shannon's entropy. In this work, the role of the SGO is to continuously adjust the image threshold value till the Shannon's entropy is maximized. The results attained with SGO + Shannon's based threshold for Th = 2 and Th-3 is presented in Figure 4.8 (a) and (b) and this results confirms that the proposed technique works well on the greyscale and the RGB scale images.

Advantages: This approach provides better image enhancement compared to other procedures and present the best values of the image quality measures than the Otsu.

Limitations: Implementation and identification of the maximized threshold is quite complex compared to the Otsu.

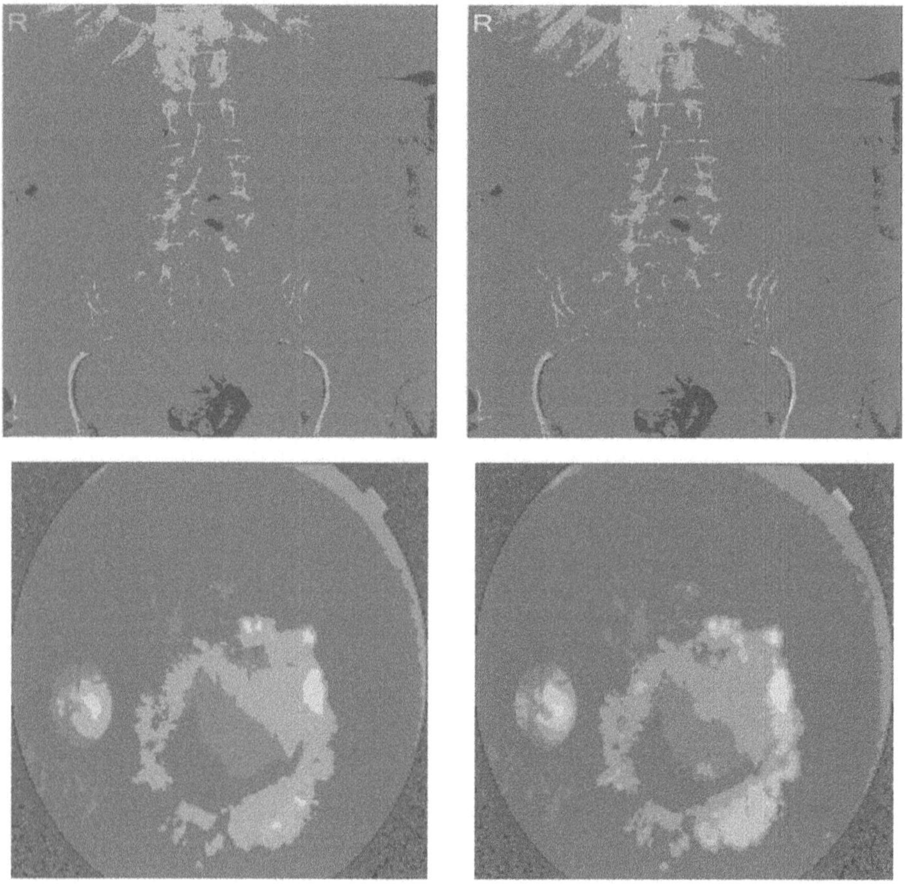

FIGURE 4.8 Shannon's entropy based bi-level and tri-level thresholding

4.4 ENTROPY BASED FEATURES IN IMAGE PROCESSING

In the literature, entropy-based thresholding methodologies are widely executed to identify a class of disease with a developed computerised system. In medical image examination, we are mainly interested in analysing the abnormalities present in the medical images with a visual check or computerised assessment. Entropy is also known as the abnormality and hence, entropy-based thresholding procedures work well on a class of medical pictures. The earlier works related with the entropy assisted thresholding of the medical images can be found in (Rajinikanth et al., 2017) and these works confirms the superiority of the entropy-based technique compared with the non-entropy technique. This section further presents the results on few chosen medical images to confirm the performance of the entropy supported enhancement scheme. The choice of a particular entropy function depends mainly on the type of the image and expertise of the operator who develops the computer algorithm.

This section presents the evaluation of a lung CT scan slice associated with the COVID-19 infection. The essential images are collected from the benchmark dataset available in (Rajinikanth et al., 2020; 2020a; Kadry et al., 2020). This database consist 20 patient's images collected using the clinical protocol and every image is available in the form of 3D. Initially, the 3D to 2D conversion is performed using the ITK-snap software and the attained slice is then resized and processed. The various procedures implemented in the proposed system is depicted in Figure 4.9.

The essential section and the related image processing procedures implemented on a chosen image with the proposed approach is clearly presented and in this study, the results attained for the lung CT scan images with COVID-19 infection is presented. Figure 4.9 depicts a framework to extract and evaluate the COVID-19 infection section using thresholding entropy-based thresholding. Initially, the patient with the COVID-19 infection is screened using the CT scan methodology, which offers a reconstructed 3D image of the lung section. The examination of 3D image is computationally complex and time consuming. Hence, 3D to 2D conversion is executed using ITK-snap (Yushkevich et al., 2016, 2016a). In this work, the axial-view of the CT scan Slice (CTS) is considered for the assessment and the essential images are collected from existing benchmark database.

The CTS collected for the assessment is associated with the unwanted body parts and a threshold-filter is then employed to separate the image into ROI and the artefact. The ROI is then assessed using the proposed technique. Initially, a SGO assisted tri-level thresholding is implemented to enhance the pneumonia infection from the lungs. During this process, a detailed assessment of the thresholding approaches, such as Otsu, Kapur, Tsallis and Shannon is performed. After the thresholding, the outcome is then compared against the original test image and the essential picture quality measures, such as Root-Mean-Squared-Error (RMSE), Peak Signal-to-Noise Ratio (PSNR), Structural-Similarity-Index-Matrix (SSIM), Normalised-Cross-Correlation (NCC), Average-Difference (AD), Structural-Content (SC) and Normalised-Absolute-Error (NAE) are computed and based on these values, the performance of the thresholding technique is confirmed. After the possible enhancement, the ROI section is then extracted using a suitable post processing technique. In this work, the well-known Distance-Regularised-Level-Set (DRLS) with a single-well technique discussed in (Sethian 1993; Li et al., 2010) is adopted and the essential ROI is then extracted. The DRLS is a semi-automated segmentation approach works based on a bounding-box technique and extracts the pixel of interest using an adaptable curve, which converges based on the increased iteration. After extracting the essential section from the thresholded image, a comparison with the Ground-Truth (GT) is executed and the essential measures, such as Jaccard, dice (F1-Score), accuracy, precision, sensitivity, specificity are computed. The post-processing eminence can be confirmed based on the values of the Jaccard, dice and the segmentation accuracy value. The experimental investigation confirms that, proposed approach helps to achieve a better outcome when Kapur's entropy assisted thresholding is implemented to pre-process the test image. This confirms that the entropy-based approach works well on the lung CTS compared to the considered non-entropy (Otsu) approach.

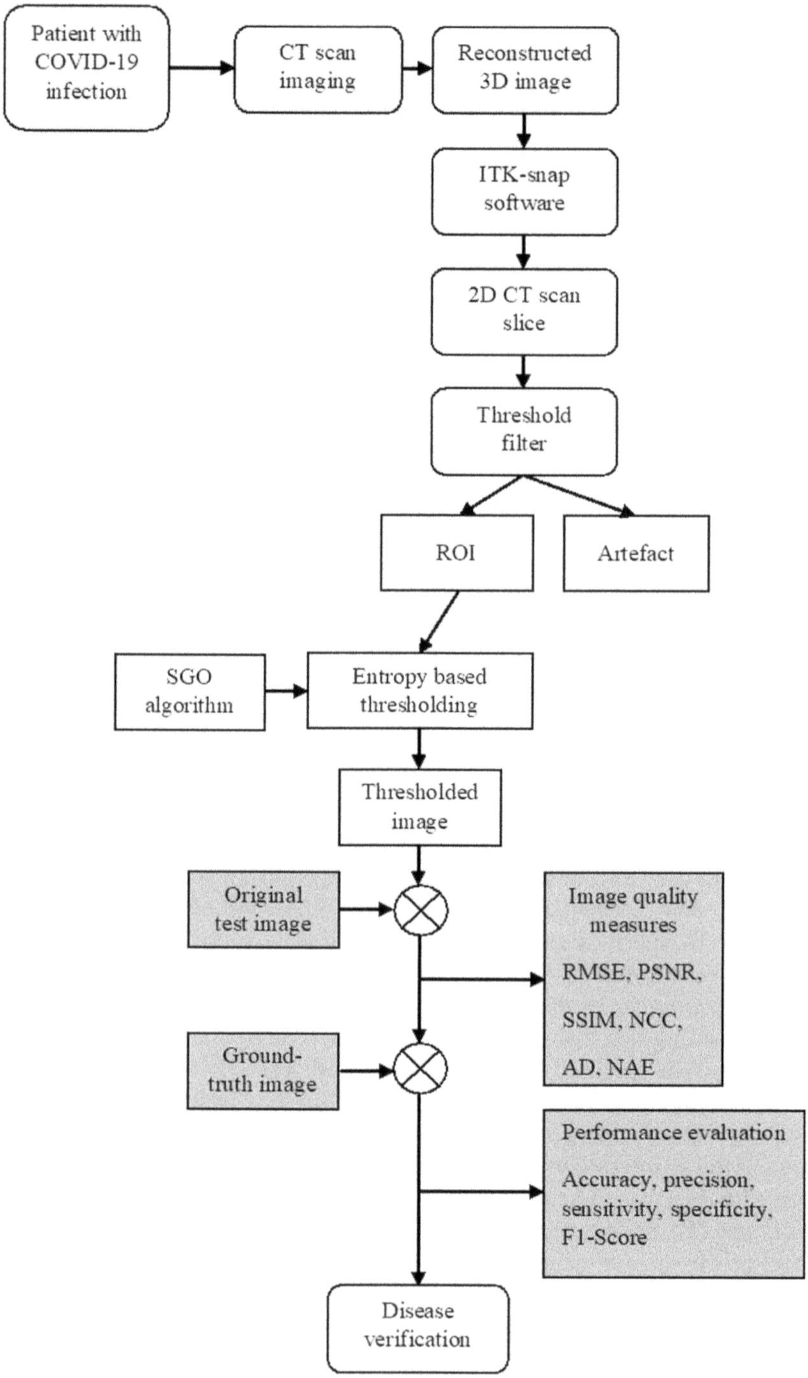

FIGURE 4.9 Traditional medical image processing procedure implemented for the lung CT scan image analysis

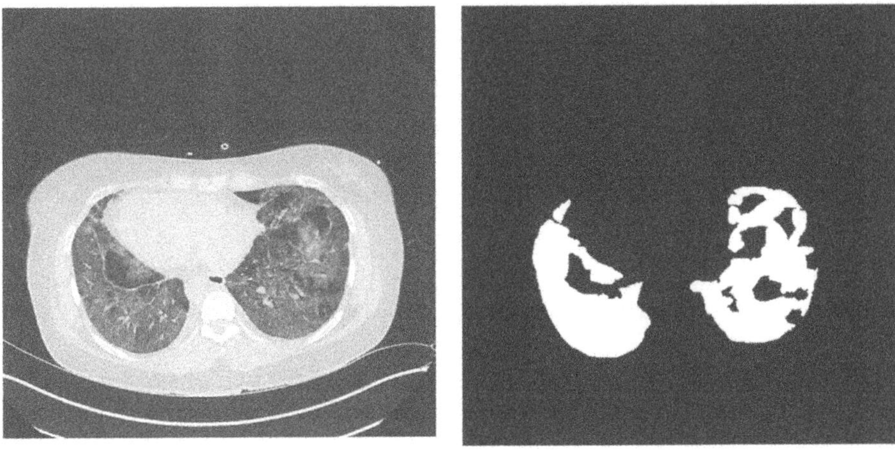

(a) Test image (b) Ground-truth

FIGURE 4.10 Sample test image and the related GT

Figure 4.10 depicts the sample test image of dimension 256x256x1 pixel collected from the benchmark COVID-19 dataset along with its GT. This dataset consists of the essential information to test the developed image processing based disease detection system. The considered test image is also depicted in Figure 4.11 (a) is then passed through a thresholding filter in order to separate the image into two sections, such as ROI as in Figure 4.11 (b) and artefact as depicted in Figure 4.11 (c). The essential information on the threshold filter can be accessed from [41–43]. After the separation, the artefact is eliminated and the ROI is then considered for the further assessment.

The considered ROI (Figure 4.11(b)) is then pre-processed using the SGO algorithm along with the chosen thresholding technique. The results attained with Otsu, Kapur, Tsallis and Shannon methods are presented in Figure 4.12 and this result confirms that, the tri-level thresholding (Th = 3) will help to enhance the visibility of

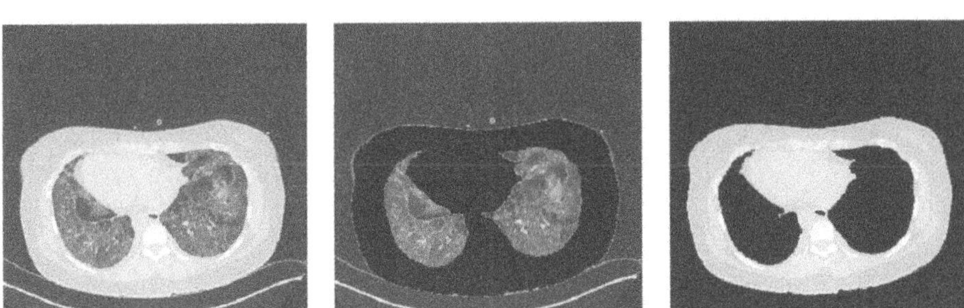

(a) Test image (b) ROI (c) Artefact

FIGURE 4.11 Results attained with the threshold filter

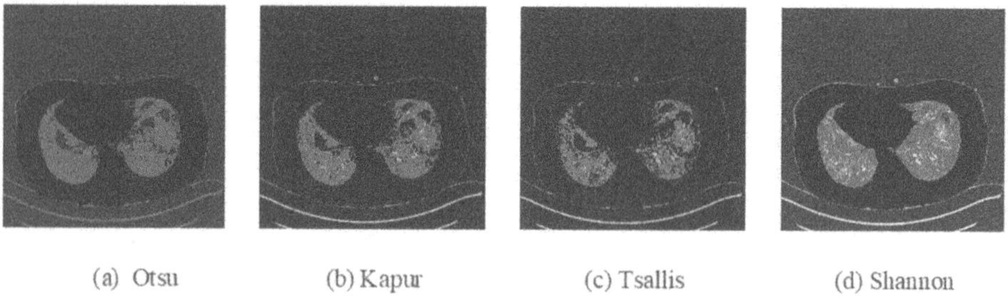

FIGURE 4.12 SGO based thresholding result attained for a chosen threshold value (Th = 3)

the ROI considerably. After enhancing the visibility of the ROI, the picture quality measures are to be computed by comparing the thresholded image with the original picture and this information can be found in the earlier works (Ponomarenko et al., 2008; Hore and Ziou, 2010).

The essential quality measures considered in this work is presented below:

$$RMSE_{(R,T)} = \sqrt{MSE_{(R,T)}} = \sqrt{\frac{1}{XY}\sum_{i=1}^{X}\sum_{j=1}^{Y}[R_{(i,j)} - T_{(i,j)}]^2} \tag{4.18}$$

$$\text{PSNR}_{(R,T)} = 20\log_{10}\left(\frac{255}{\sqrt{MSE_{(R,T)}}}\right);\text{dB} \tag{4.19}$$

$$\text{SSIM}_{(R,T)} = \frac{1}{M}\sum_{z=1}^{M} SSIM_{(Rz,Tz)} \tag{4.20}$$

$$\text{NAE}_{(R,T)} = \frac{\sum_{i=1}^{X}\sum_{j=1}^{Y}|R_{(i,j)} - T_{(i,j)}|}{\sum_{i=1}^{X}\sum_{j=1}^{Y}|R_{(i,j)}|} \tag{4.21}$$

$$\text{NCC}_{(R,T)} = \frac{\sum_{i=1}^{X}\sum_{j=1}^{Y} R_{(i,j)} \cdot T_{(i,j)}}{\sum_{i=1}^{X}\sum_{j=1}^{Y} R^2_{(i,j)}} \tag{4.22}$$

$$\text{AD}_{(R,T)} = \frac{\sum_{i=1}^{X}\sum_{j=1}^{Y} R_{(i,j)} - T_{(i,j)}}{XY} \tag{4.23}$$

$$SC(R,T) = \frac{\sum_{i=1}^{X}\sum_{j=1}^{Y} R^2_{(i,j)}}{\sum_{i=1}^{X}\sum_{j=1}^{Y} T^2_{(i,j)}} \tag{4.24}$$

where, R_z and T_z are the image contents at the z-th local window; and M is the number of local windows in the image.

In all the expressions, $X *Y$ is the size of considered image, R is the original test image and S is the segmented image of a chosen threshold.

Figures 4.13 and 4.14 presents the essential information attained with the thresholding process and this result confirms that, the Shannon's entropy thresholding offers superior result.

Table 4.1 depicts the essential information computed with the proposed comparative study. This table confirms that the RMSE, PSNR and SSIM attained with the Shannon's thresholding is superior compared to the Otsu and other entropy assisted techniques. The SSIM-map presented in Figure 4.13 also confirms that, the correlation between the test image and the thresholded image in Shannon's technique is better compared to the alternative methods.

After the thresholding, a chosen segmentation (DRLS) is then implemented to extract the ROI and the attained results are depicted in Figure 4.15. Figure 4.15 (a) depicts the initial bounding-box initiated by the operator to extract the ROI and Figure 4.15 (b) presents the converged bounding-box in a 3D view. The converged DRLS for the Otsu and Tsallis enhanced images are presented in Figure 4.15 (c) and (d) respectively. Even though, it is a semi-automated segmentation technique, it helps to extract the infected lungs with better accuracy. Similar procedure is implemented on the Kapur and the Shannon thresholded images and the attained results are considered for the further assessment.

Figure 4.16 (a) to (d) depicts the DRLS segmented ROI from the lung CTS and these results confirms that, the proposed methodology helps to extract the infected section with greater accuracy. After extracting the ROI, every RO is then compared against the GT and the essential information then computed to confirm the superiority of the chosen thresholding and segmentation procedure. The results attained with

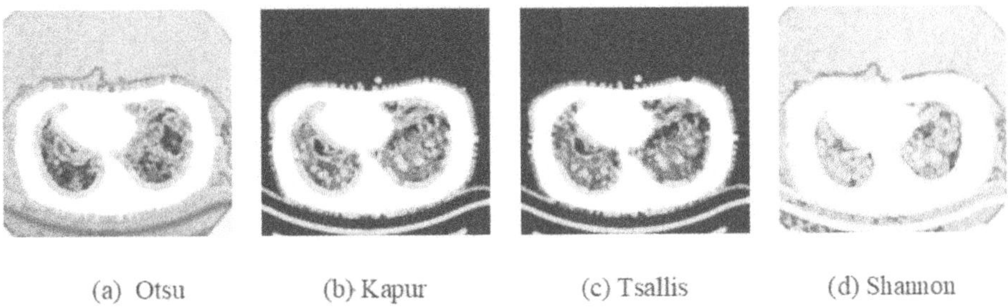

FIGURE 4.13 SSIM map during the image comparison

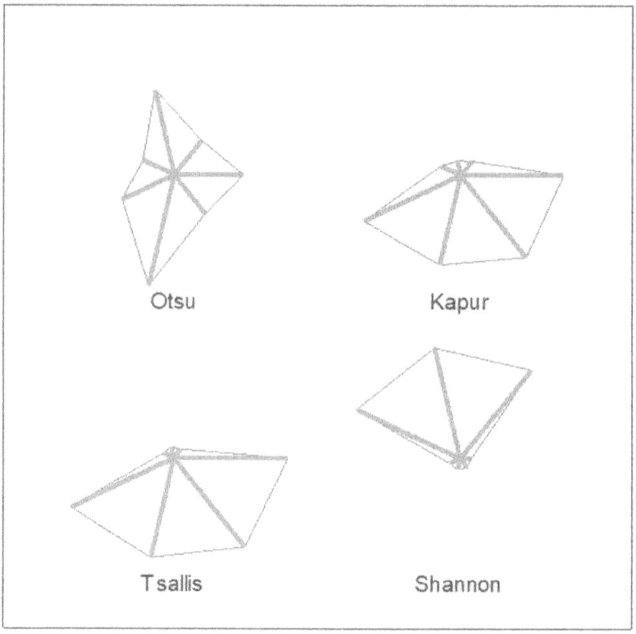

FIGURE 4.14 Glyph-plot to confirm the overall performance of the thresholding technique

the proposed comparative assessment can be found in Table 4.2. This table also confirms that the segmentation accuracy and the Jaccard and dice values attained with the Kapur's entropy assisted method is better compared to the alternatives.

The essential values presented in Table 4.2 are computed using the following measures:

$$Jaccard = \frac{GTI \cap SI}{GTI \cup SI} = \frac{TP}{TP + FP + FN} \tag{4.25}$$

$$Dice = F1\ Score = \frac{2|GTI \cap SI|}{|GTI| + |SI|} = \frac{2TP}{2TP + FP + FN} \tag{4.26}$$

TABLE 4.1
Image Quality Measures Computed Using Thresholded Image

Method	RMSE	PSNR	SSIM	NCC	AD	SC	NAE
Otsu	25.3665	20.0456	0.7560	0.5629	16.1266	2.8838	0.4306
Kapur	33.0761	17.7405	0.4281	0.5097	26.0148	2.5297	0.6945
Tsallis	35.5474	17.1146	0.4095	0.4685	27.5876	2.6940	0.7365
Shannon	12.3702	26.2832	0.8758	0.8845	6.8750	1.2171	0.2448

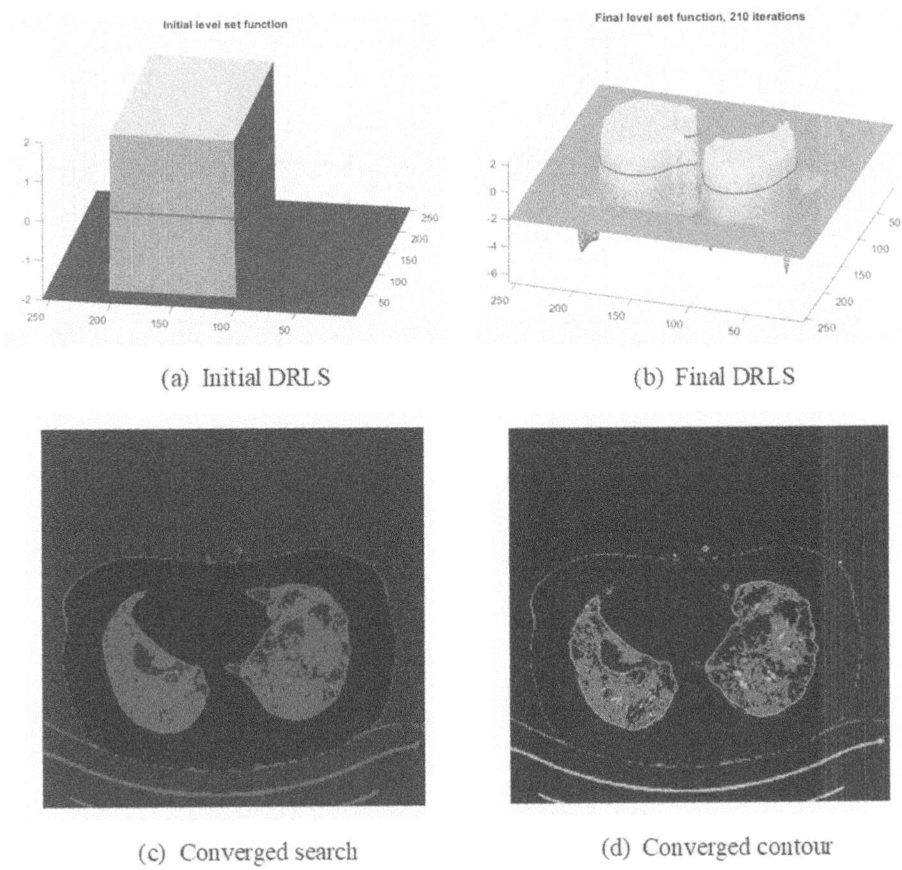

(a) Initial DRLS (b) Final DRLS

(c) Converged search (d) Converged contour

FIGURE 4.15 Results attained with the DRLS segmentation on the chosen test image

$$Accuracy = \frac{TP + TN}{TP + TN + FP + FN} \tag{4.27}$$

$$Precision = \frac{TP}{TP + FP} \tag{4.28}$$

$$Sensitivity = \frac{TP}{TP + FN} \tag{4.29}$$

$$Specificity = \frac{TN}{TN + FP} \tag{4.30}$$

$$NPV = \frac{TN}{TN + FN} \tag{4.31}$$

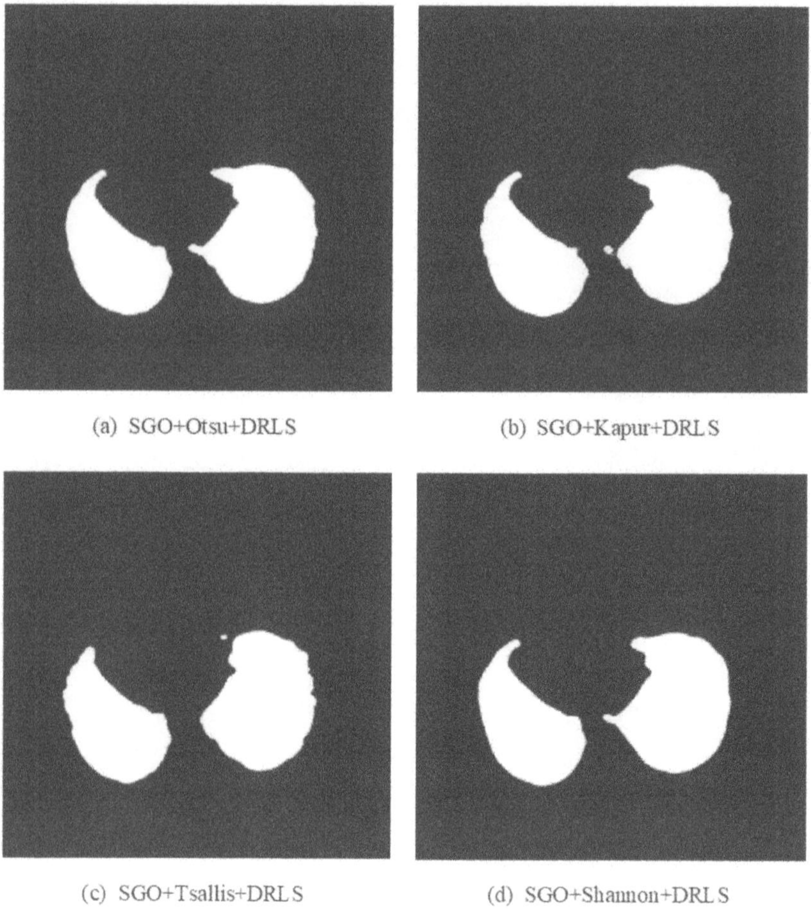

FIGURE 4.16 Segmentation outcome attained with the DRLS technique

TABLE 4.2
Image Performance Measures Attained With the DRLS Segmentation

Method	TP	TN	FP	FN	Jaccard	Dice	Accuracy	Precision	Sensitivity	Specificity
Otsu	2781	56281	79	1121	69.86	82.25	98.01	97.23	71.27	99.85
Kapur	2774	56414	86	1024	71.42	83.33	98.16	96.99	73.04	99.85
Tsallis	2735	56574	125	1028	70.34	82.59	98.09	95.63	72.68	99.78
Shannon	2770	56400	90	1044	70.95	83.01	98.12	96.85	72.63	99.84

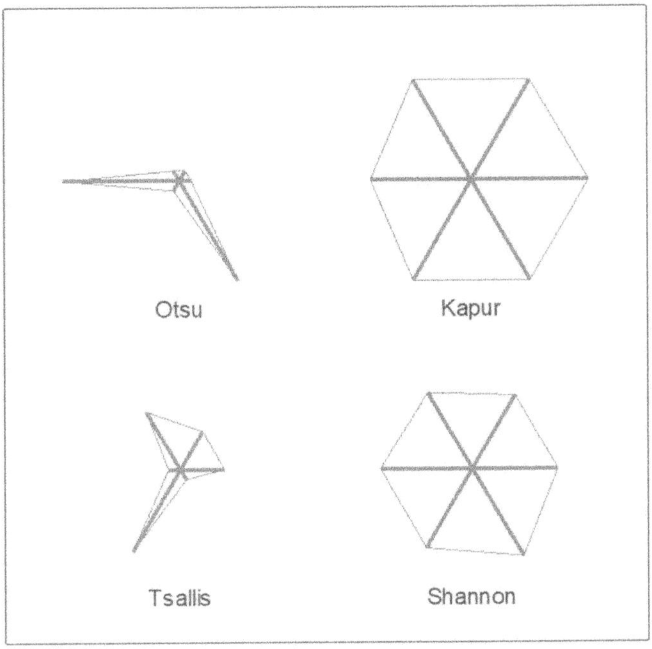

FIGURE 4.17 Glyph-plot to confirm the overall performance of the proposed technique

where *GTI* is the ground-truth-image, *SI* is the segmented image, *TP*, *TN*, *FP* and *FN* denotes true-positive, true-negative, false-positive and false-negative, respectively.

The overall superiority of the proposed method is also confirmed using a Glyph-plot depicted in Figure 4.17 and this figure also confirms that the performance of the Kapur is better compared to Otsu, Tsallis and Shannon. All the above said results confirm that the entropy-based methods can offer superior results when a medical grade images are processed. The processed medical grade images are then considered to examine the disease with better accuracy. When a feature extraction and the classification section is included in the proposed approach depicted in Figure 4.9, then the whole system can be considered as a machine-learning system to detect the COVID-19 infection using the lung CTS.

4.5 SUMMARY

This section of the book presented information regarding the thresholding of the greyscale and RGB scale pictures using the bi-level and tri-level thresholding. The thresholding procedures with the entropy and non-entropy procedures with a chosen technique are clearly discussed with appropriate results. The need for the image thresholding procedure for the medical images is discussed in brief and the commonly implemented procedures, such as Otsu, Kapur, Tsallis and

Shannon are considered to pre-process the considered test images. In this work, the SGO assisted technique is adopted to enhance the test image with a chosen pre-processing technique. From this section also presented the assessment of the lung CTS of COVID-19 infected person. The essential thresholding is implemented using the SGO and a selected pre-processing technique and the extraction of the ROI is implemented using the DRLS segmentation. The performance of the pre-processing and segmentation techniques are evaluated using the commonly used approaches and this result confirmed that, the entropy-based technique helps to attain better result compared to other methods. A detailed framework is also suggested to evaluate the COVID-19 infection and the attained result helped to reach better values of the Jaccard, dice and segmentation accuracy. In future, the proposed framework can be used along with the feature extraction and the classification methods to implement a scheme for the automated evaluate of the COVID-19 infection from lung CTS.

REFERENCES

Acharya, U. R., Fernandes, S. L., WeiKoh, J. E., Ciaccio, E. J., Fabell, M. K. M., Tanik, U. J., & Yeong, C. H. (2019). Automated detection of Alzheimer's disease using brain MRI images–a study with various feature extraction techniques. *Journal of Medical Systems*, 43(9), 302.

Balan, N. S., Kumar, A. S., Raja, N. S. M., & Rajinikanth, V. (2016). Optimal multilevel image thresholding to improve the visibility of Plasmodium sp. in blood smear images. In *Proceedings of the International Conference on Soft Computing Systems* (pp. 563–571). Springer.

Dey, N., Rajinikanth, V., Ashour, A. S., & Tavares, J. M. R. (2018). Social group optimization supported segmentation and evaluation of skin melanoma images. *Symmetry*, 10(2), 51.

Dey, N., Rajinikanth, V., Shi, F., Tavares, J. M. R., Moraru, L., Karthik, K. A., & Emmanuel, C. (2019). Social-Group-Optimization based tumor evaluation tool for clinical brain MRI of Flair/diffusion-weighted modality. *Biocybernetics and Biomedical Engineering*, 39(3), 843–856.

Dey, N., Shi, F., & Rajinikanth, V. (2020). Image examination system to detect gastric polyps from endoscopy images. *Information Technology and Intelligent Transportation Systems*, 323, 107–116.

Fang, J., Zheng, H., Liu, J., Zhao, J., Zhang, Y., & Wang, K. (2018). A transformer fault diagnosis model using an optimal hybrid dissolved gas analysis features subset with improved social group optimization-support vector machine classifier. *Energies*, 11(8), 1922.

Feng, X., Wang, Y., Yu, H., & Luo, F. (2016). A novel intelligence algorithm based on the social group optimization behaviors. *IEEE Transactions on systems, man, and cybernetics: systems*, 48(1), 65–76.

Feng, Y., Zhao, H., Li, X., Zhang, X., & Li, H. (2017). A multi-scale 3D Otsu thresholding algorithm for medical image segmentation. *Digital Signal Processing*, *60*, 186–199.

Fernandes, S. L., Rajinikanth, V., & Kadry, S. (2019). A hybrid framework to evaluate breast abnormality using infrared thermal images. *IEEE Consumer Electronics Magazine*, 8(5), 31–36.

Fernandes, S. L., Tanik, U. J., Rajinikanth, V., & Karthik, K. A. (2019a). A reliable framework for accurate brain image examination and treatment planning based on early diagnosis support for clinicians. *Neural Computing and Applications*, 1–12.

Hore, A., & Ziou, D. (2010). Image quality metrics: PSNR vs. SSIM. In *2010 20th international conference on pattern recognition* (pp. 2366–2369). IEEE.

Kadry, S., Rajinikanth, V., Rho, S., Raja, N. S. M., Rao, V. S., & Thanaraj, K. P. (2020). Development of a Machine-Learning System to Classify Lung CT Scan Images into Normal/COVID-19 Class. *arXiv preprint arXiv:2004.13122.*

Kapur, J. N., & Kesavan, H. K. (1992). Entropy optimization principles and their applications. In *Entropy and energy dissipation in water resources* (pp. 3). Springer.

Kapur, J. N., Sahoo, P. K., & Wong, A. K. (1985). A new method for gray-level picture thresholding using the entropy of the histogram. *Computer vision, graphics, and image processing*, 29(3), 273–285.

Lakshmi, V. S., Tebby, S. G., Shriranjani, D., & Rajinikanth, V. (2016). Chaotic cuckoo search and Kapur/Tsallis approach in segmentation of T. Cruzi from blood smear images. *International Journal of Computer Science and Information Security (IJCSIS), 14,* 51–56.

Li, C., Xu, C., Gui, C., & Fox, M. D.(2010). Distance regularized level set evolution and its application to image segmentation. *IEEE transactions on image processing*, 19(12), 3243–3254.

Li, Y., Jiao, L., Shang, R., & Stolkin, R. (2015). Dynamic-context cooperative quantum-behaved particle swarm optimization based on multilevel thresholding applied to medical image segmentation. *Information Sciences*, *294*, 408–422.

Lin, J. (1991). Divergence measures based on the Shannon entropy. *IEEE Transactions on Information Theory*, 37(1), 145–151.

Manic, K. S., Priya, R. K., & Rajinikanth, V. (2016). Image multithresholding based on Kapur/Tsallis entropy and firefly algorithm. *Indian Journal of Science and Technology*, 9(12), 89949.

Manikandan, S., Ramar, K., Iruthayarajan, M. W., & Srinivasagan, K. G. (2014). Multilevel thresholding for segmentation of medical brain images using real coded genetic algorithm. *Measurement*, *47*, 558–568.

Monisha, R., Mrinalini, R., Britto, M. N., Ramakrishnan, R., & Rajinikanth, V. (2019). Social group optimization and Shannon's function-based RGB image multi-level thresholding. In *Smart Intelligent Computing and Applications* (pp. 123). Springer.

Naik, A., Satapathy, S. C., Ashour, A. S., & Dey, N. (2018). Social group optimization for global optimization of multimodal functions and data clustering problems. *Neural Computing and Applications*, 30(1), 271–287.

Otsu, N. (1979). A threshold selection method from gray-level histograms. *IEEE Transactions on Systems, Man, and Cybernetics*, 9(1), 62–66.

Plastino, A. R., & Plastino, A. (1993). Stellar polytropes and Tsallis' entropy. *Physics Letters A*, 174(5-6), 384–386.

Ponomarenko, N., Lukin, V., Egiazarian, K., Astola, J., Carli, M., & Battisti, F. (2008). Color image database for evaluation of image quality metrics. In *2008 IEEE 10th workshop on multimedia signal processing* (pp. 403–408). IEEE.

Praveen, S. P., Rao, K. T., & Janakiramaiah, B. (2018). Effective allocation of resources and task scheduling in cloud environment using social group optimization. *Arabian Journal for Science and Engineering*, 43(8), 4265–4272.

Pugalenthi, R., Rajakumar, M. P., Ramya, J., & Rajinikanth, V. (2019). Evaluation and classification of the brain tumor MRI using machine learning technique. *Journal of Control Engineering and Applied Informatics*, 21(4), 12–21.

Raguram, N., Rahul, R., Raghul, C., & Sankaran, D. (2018). Noise Tainted RGB Image Thresholding by Integrating SGO and Kapur's Function. In *2018 International Conference on Recent Trends in Electrical, Control and Communication (RTECC)* (pp. 19–22). IEEE.

Raja, N. S. M., Fernandes, S. L., Dey, N., Satapathy, S. C., & Rajinikanth, V. (2018). Contrast enhanced medical MRI evaluation using Tsallis entropy and region growing segmentation. *Journal of Ambient Intelligence and Humanized Computing*, 1–12.

Raja, N. S. M., Rajinikanth, V., Fernandes, S. L., & Satapathy, S. C. (2017). Segmentation of breast thermal images using Kapur's entropy and hidden Markov random field. *Journal of Medical Imaging and Health Informatics*, 7(8), 1825–1829.

Rajinikanth, V., & Couceiro, M. S. (2015). Optimal multilevel image threshold selection using a novel objective function. In *Information Systems Design and Intelligent Applications* (pp. 177). Springer.

Rajinikanth, V., & Couceiro, M. S. (2015a). RGB histogram based color image segmentation using firefly algorithm. *Procedia Computer Science, 46*, 1449–1457.

Rajinikanth, V., & Satapathy, S. C. (2018). Segmentation of ischemic stroke lesion in brain MRI based on social group optimization and Fuzzy-Tsallis entropy. *Arabian Journal for Science and Engineering*, 43(8), 4365–4378.

Rajinikanth, V., Dey, N., Kavallieratou, E., & Lin, H. (2020). Firefly algorithm-based Kapur's thresholding and Hough transform to extract leukocyte section from hematological images. In *Applications of Firefly Algorithm and its Variants* (pp. 221). Springer.

Rajinikanth, V., Dey, N., Raj, A. N. J., Hassanien, A. E., Santosh, K. C., & Raja, N. (2020). Harmony-search and otsu based system for coronavirus disease (COVID-19) detection using lung CT scan images. *arXiv preprint arXiv:2004.03431.*

Rajinikanth, V., Kadry, S., Thanaraj, K. P., Kamalanand, K., & Seo, S. (2020b). Firefly-Algorithm Supported Scheme to Detect COVID-19 Lesion in Lung CT Scan Images using Shannon Entropy and Markov-Random-Field. *arXiv preprint arXiv:2004.09239.*

Rajinikanth, V., Madhavaraja, N., Satapathy, S. C., & Fernandes, S. L. (2017). Otsu's multithresholding and active contour snake model to segment dermoscopy images. *Journal of Medical Imaging and Health Informatics*, 7(8), 1837–1840.

Rajinikanth, V., Raja, N. S. M., & Kamalanand, K. (2017). Firefly algorithm assisted segmentation of tumor from brain MRI using Tsallis function and Markov random field. *Journal of Control Engineering and Applied Informatics*, 19(3), 97–106.

Rajinikanth, V., Satapathy, S. C., Dey, N., & Lin, H. (2018). Evaluation of ischemic stroke region from CT/MR images using hybrid image processing techniques. In *Intelligent Multidimensional Data and Image Processing* (pp. 194–219). IGI Global.

Roopini, I. T., Vasanthi, M., Rajinikanth, V., Rekha, M., & Sangeetha, M. (2018). Segmentation of tumor from brain MRI using fuzzy entropy and distance regularised level set. In *Computational Signal Processing and Analysis* (pp. 297). Springer.

Satapathy, S. C., Raja, N. S. M., Rajinikanth, V., Ashour, A. S., & Dey, N. (2018). Multilevel image thresholding using Otsu and chaotic bat algorithm. *Neural Computing and Applications*, 29(12), 1285–1307.

Satapathy, S., & Naik, A. (2016). Social group optimization (SGO): a new population evolutionary optimization technique. *Complex & Intelligent Systems*, 2(3), 173–203.

Sethian, J. A. (1996). A fast marching level set method for monotonically advancing fronts. *Proceedings of the National Academy of Sciences*, 93(4), 1591–1595.

Shree, T. V., Revanth, K., Raja, N. S. M., & Rajinikanth, V. (2018). A hybrid image processing approach to examine abnormality in retinal optic disc. *Procedia Computer Science, 125*, 157–164.

Shriranjani, D., Tebby, S. G., Satapathy, S. C., Dey, N., & Rajinikanth, V. (2018). Kapur's entropy and active contour-based segmentation and analysis of retinal optic disc. In *Computational Signal Processing and Analysis* (pp. 287). Springer.

Wu, Y., Zhou, Y., Saveriades, G., Agaian, S., Noonan, J. P., & Natarajan, P. (2013). Local Shannon entropy measure with statistical tests for image randomness. *Information Sciences, 222*, 323–342.

Yushkevich, P. A., Gao, Y., & Gerig, G. (2016). ITK-SNAP: An interactive tool for semi-automatic segmentation of multi-modality biomedical images. In *2016 38th Annual International Conference of the IEEE Engineering in Medicine and Biology Society (EMBC)* (pp. 3342–3345). IEEE.

Yushkevich, P. A., Piven, J., Hazlett, H. C., Smith, R. G., Ho, S., Gee, J. C., & Gerig, G. (2006a). User-guided 3D active contour segmentation of anatomical structures: significantly improved efficiency and reliability. *Neuroimage*, 31(3), 1116–1128.

5 Case Studies With Medical Imaging

In medical field, diseases recognition by computerized and semi-automated analytic scheme plays a chief position during treatment planning and implementation. The computer software developed to identify disease based on the medical images that are recorded by means of a specific modality, which further act as a supporting arrangement for the disease forecast. Execution of an appropriate diagnosis scheme would considerably decrease the burden of the doctors who are involved in the disease detection process. Image appraisal based on the preferred computer algorithm is gaining reputation due to its accuracy and adaptability to a selection of images with varied dimension and orientation. Throughout the medical image assessment, the extraction and evaluation of the infected division using an appropriate procedure is largely implemented to examine the greyscale and RGB images (Rezatofighi and Soltanian-Zadeh, 2011; Manickavasagam et al., 2014; Lakshmi et al., 2016; Balan et al., 2016; Dey et al., 2019; Chaki and Dey, 2020; Bhandary et al., 2020; Rajinikanth et al., 2020).

The thresholding and segmentation is frequently used image pre-processing and post-processing techniques to enhance and extract a particular section (ROI) from the image. Usually, a substantial amount of the ROI mining practices are existing in the literature and based on the implementation, it can be classified as; (i) Automated segmentation and (ii) Semi-automated segmentation techniques and the choice of a particular practice depends on the expertise of the operator and the complexity of the test image; which is to be examined (Jesline et al., 2020). The remaining part of this chapter clearly presents the medical image processing procedures adopted for a class of image modalities (Raja et al., 2015; Fernandes et al., 2019; Rajinikanth et al., 2020; Dey et al., 2020). In this work, a brief over view of the medical image assessment techniques are presented to evaluate the abnormalities in eye, brain, lung and the breast section and for the breast assessment, a machine-learning assisted detection is also discussed in brief. For the simplicity, this work considered the SGO algorithm assisted Shannon's entropy-based thresholding scheme to pre-process the considered medical grade images in order to enhance the infected section (ROI). The extraction of the chosen section is achieved using the preferred segmentation procedures, such as DRLS (Li et al., 2005), active contour (Kass et al., 1988; Cohen, 1991), watershed (Shafarenko et al., 1997; Nguyen et al., 2003) and Seed-Region-Growing (SRG) (Mehnert and Jackway, 1997; Xu and Cumming, 1999) based methods. For the considered image category, feature extraction with the Gray Level Co-occurrence Matrix (GLCM) can be implemented to mine the vital image information and finally the disease classification can be achieved by employing a binary classifier.

5.1 MEDICAL IMAGE MODALITIES

In the medical domain, the disease in the internal and external body organs are widely assessed with the help of the images recorded using a prescribed protocol. The disease in a chosen organ is commonly recorded non-invasively using a chosen imaging modalities. In the literature, a number of modalities are available to record the condition of the organ and in this work, the commonly used image modalities, such as digital fundus image (eye disease assessment), MRI (brain abnormality assessment), and thermal imaging (breast condition assessment) are considered for the study. Every modality has its merit and the image examination system (pre-processing and post-processing) proposed for a chosen modality will work on other images and provides the necessary results.

5.2 FUNDUS IMAGE EXAMINATION

Eye is one of the vital sensory organs in human physiology and the abnormality in the eye will severely disturb the decision-making capacity of the brain. The performance of the eye degrades due to various reasons and the aging is one of the chief reasons. In this section, the detection of the common eye disease called the Glaucoma is presented and the condition of the eye (healthy/Glaucoma) is confirmed by computing the optic-cup to optic-disc ratio. To achieve this, the well-known Fundus Retinal Image (FRI) database called the RIM-ONE is considered for the assessment (Fumero et al., 2011; Sivaswamy et al., 2015).

The stages involved in the assessment of cup-disc ration are depicted in Figure 5.1 and this technique is separately executed for the cup and the disc. Initially, the digital FRI is pre-processed using the SGO and the Shannon's entropy-based technique with a chosen Th = 3. After enhancing the FRI, the essential ROI (cup/disc) is extracted using the DRLS segmentation. Then the extracted section is converted into binary and the essential pixel values are computed. The ratio between the cup and disc pixel is then computed and based on its value, the Glaucoma is confirmed.

5.2.1 Pre-processing

The pre-processing is one of the generally adopted image augmentation procedure to separate the ROI from the background. In this work, the SGO and Shannon's

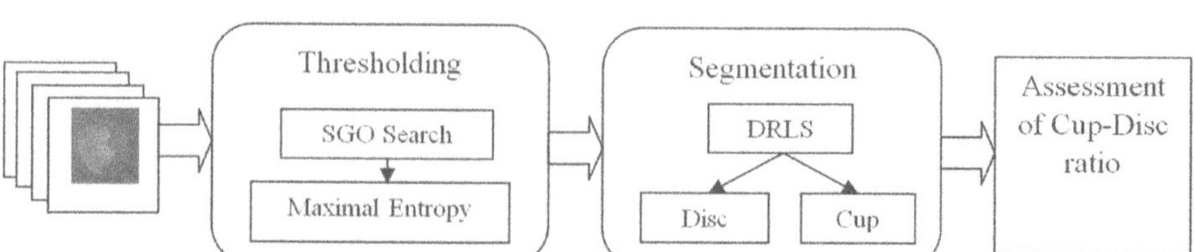

FIGURE 5.1 Block diagram of the Glaucoma detection using the retinal image

entropy-based thresholding is implemented and in this work, a tri-level thresholding is implemented to separate the FRI into background, ROI and other retinal section. In this method, the SGO is allowed to arbitrarily vary the RGB histogram of the FRI till the Shannon's entropy value is maximized. When maximized entropy is achieved, the search stops and the threshold image are presented as the result. The main task of the pre-processing operation is to enhance the ROI (cup and disc in FRI) based on the user's need.

5.2.2 Post-Processing

The major role of the post processing technique is to extract the ROI from the pre-processed image and in this work, the DRLS segmentation procedure is adopted as the post-processing technique, which separately extracts the binary form of the optic-cup and optic-disc from the FRI. The implemented DRLS is a semi-automated segmentation technique and it extracts the essential image region using a bounding-box (BB) initiated by the operator. When the iteration increases, the BB is allowed to shrink towards the pixel groups to be identified and extracted. In this work, a separate BB is assigned for cup as well as disc and the outcome of the DRLS segmentation is in binary form and the pixel ration of the image is then considered to separate the FRI images into normal and Glaucoma class.

5.2.3 Assessment and Validation

The remaining part of this sub-section presents the results attained with the proposed procedure on the RIM-ONE FRI database. The performance of the proposed system is assessed based on the ratio attained between the cup and disc and this ration is then considered to separate the images into two groups, such as healthy and Glaucoma.

The results attained using DRLS segmentation on a chosen FRI is depicted in Figure 5.2 After considering the test image, its ROI is then enhanced using the SGO + entropy based thresholding for Th = 3. After enhancing the ROI, its value is then mined using the DRLS technique. This DRLS is used to mine both the cup and the disc from the image using a varied BB dimension. The BB should enclose the ROI is to be extracted. In both the cases, the number of iteration is assigned as 500 and the BB is allowed to converge towards the pixel group of the disc or cup section and if the converged BB identifies all the possible pixels of the cup/disc section, then the DRLS search stops and a binary form of the extracted section is presented. The positive pixels (binary 1) are then computed using as appropriate method and finally, the ratio between the cup and disc is computed to conform the condition of the considered test image.

Figure 5.3 presents the result attained with the proposed technique on other RIM-ONE test image cases and this image also depicts the binary form of the disc and cup sections extracted using the proposed technique. This result confirms that, the implemented pre-processing and post-processing helps to attain

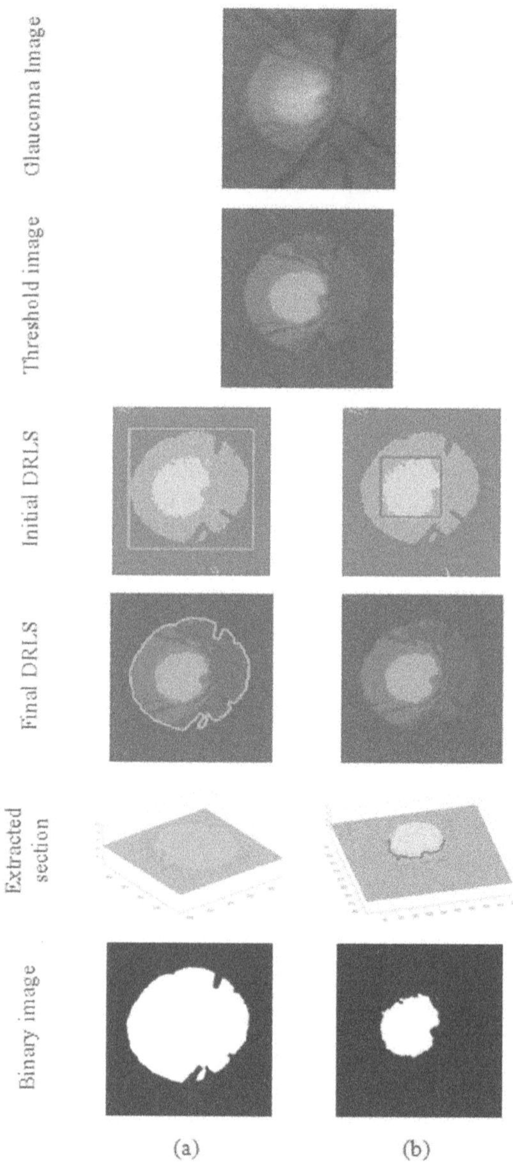

FIGURE 5.2 Assessment of the retinal image using different techniques to detect Glaucoma

better outcome on the considered FRI. The evaluation of the optic-disc and optic-cup pixels is presented in Table 5.1 along with the attained cup/disc ratio for the chosen test picture. The cup/disc ration helps to classify the FRI into normal and Glaucoma class (Sharma et al., 2008; Liu et al., 2009; Bock et al., 2010; Yu et al., 2019).

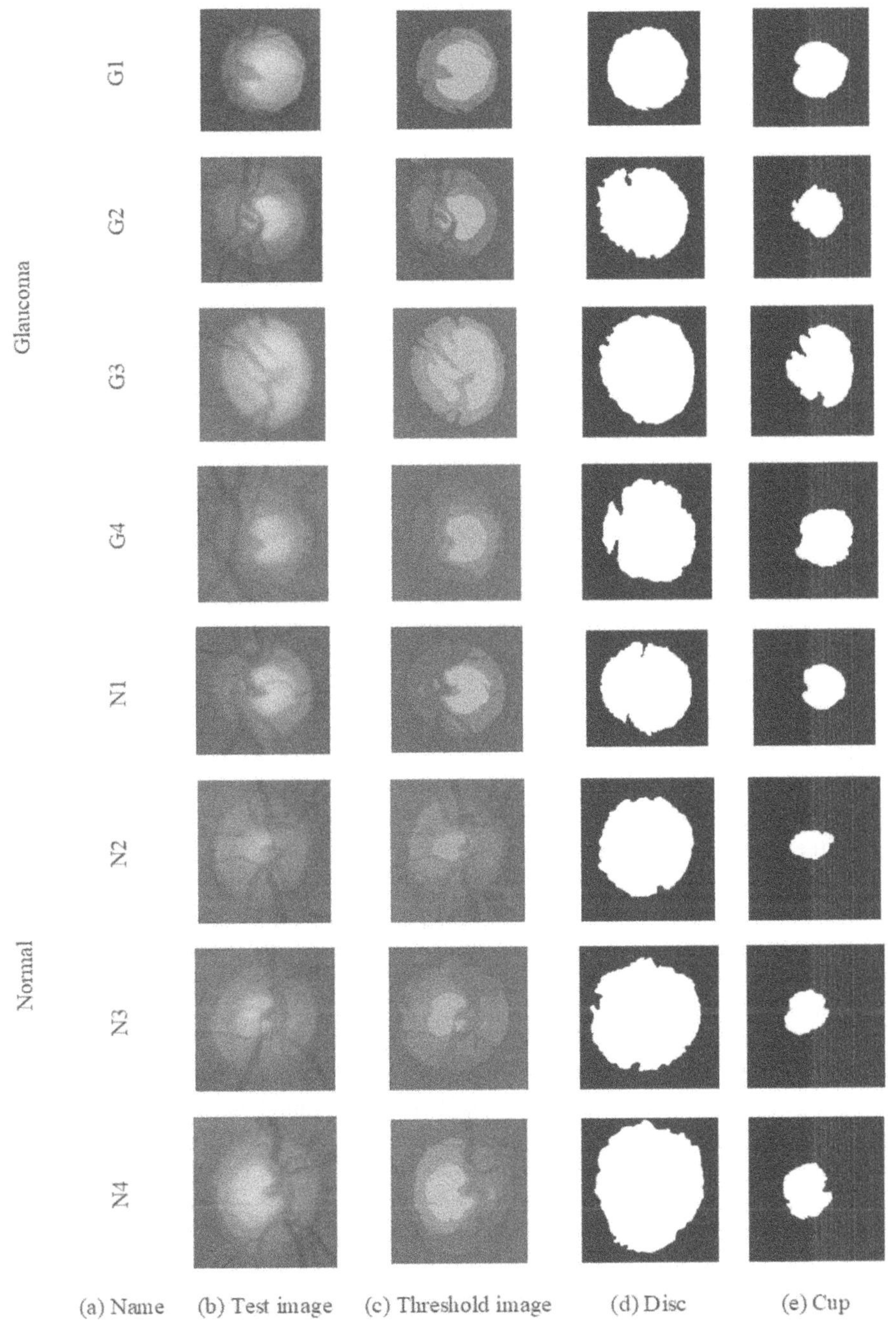

FIGURE 5.3 The results attained using sample test images are depicted with appropriate sub-sections

TABLE 5.1
Essential Pixel Level Information Attained for the Cup and Disc Sections for the Considered FRI

Class	Image	Disc pixels	Cup pixels	Cup/Disc ratio
Glaucoma	G1	55186	23817	0.4316
	G2	113550	33771	0.2974
	G3	345276	172338	0.4991
	G4	162538	60309	0.3710
Normal	N1	51859	12812	0.2471
	N2	169089	22325	0.1320
	N3	216343	33958	0.1570
	N4	327342	61189	0.1869

Similar procedure executed on the other related test images presented in Figure 5.4 and the disease in these images is identified based on the attained cup/disc ratio. Figure 5.4 (a) presents the chosen test image, Figure 5.4 (b) and (c) presents the extracted cup and disc section using the DRLS and Figure 5.4 (d) shows the attained cup/disc ration. The result of this study confirmed that, proposed technique helps to provide better result on the considered FRI dataset.

5.3 BRAIN MRI ASSESSMENT

Brain is one of the prime organs in human physiology and the disease in the brain is to be treated with care. The disease in brain will severely affect the normal behaviour of the person and the untreated brain illness will lead to death. Hence, in recent years, a number of procedures are proposed and implemented to detect the disease in brain using the medical image assisted approaches. MRI is one of the normally chosen imaging modality to examine the brain section and in this work; the MRI assisted detection of the brain abnormalities, such as stroke and tumour is performed using the benchmark datasets. In this chapter, the brain MRI of ISLES2015 (ischemic stroke) (Maier et al., 2015; 2017) and the BRATS2013 and BRATS2015 (tumour) (Menze et al., 2013; 2014; Dvořák et al., 2015) is collected from the benchmark dataset and the 3D to 2D to conversion is then implemented using the ITK-snap and then the axial-view of the 2D slice is considered for the examination. This research aims to develop a machine leering system to classify the considered MRI slices into normal/disease class using a series of procedures, such as (i) pre-processing (SGO and Shannon based thresholding), (ii) post-processing, (iii) GLCM feature extraction, (iv) Bat Algorithm based feature selection, (v) classification and validation of the attained result.

The earlier work similar to the proposed technique can be found in the earlier research works on the stroke and the tumour evaluation using SGO based technique.

Table 5.2 shows the number of images considered in the proposed work to test the proposed image processing system; which helps to detect the brain abnormalities, such as stroke and the tumour using the 2D slices of the brain MRI.

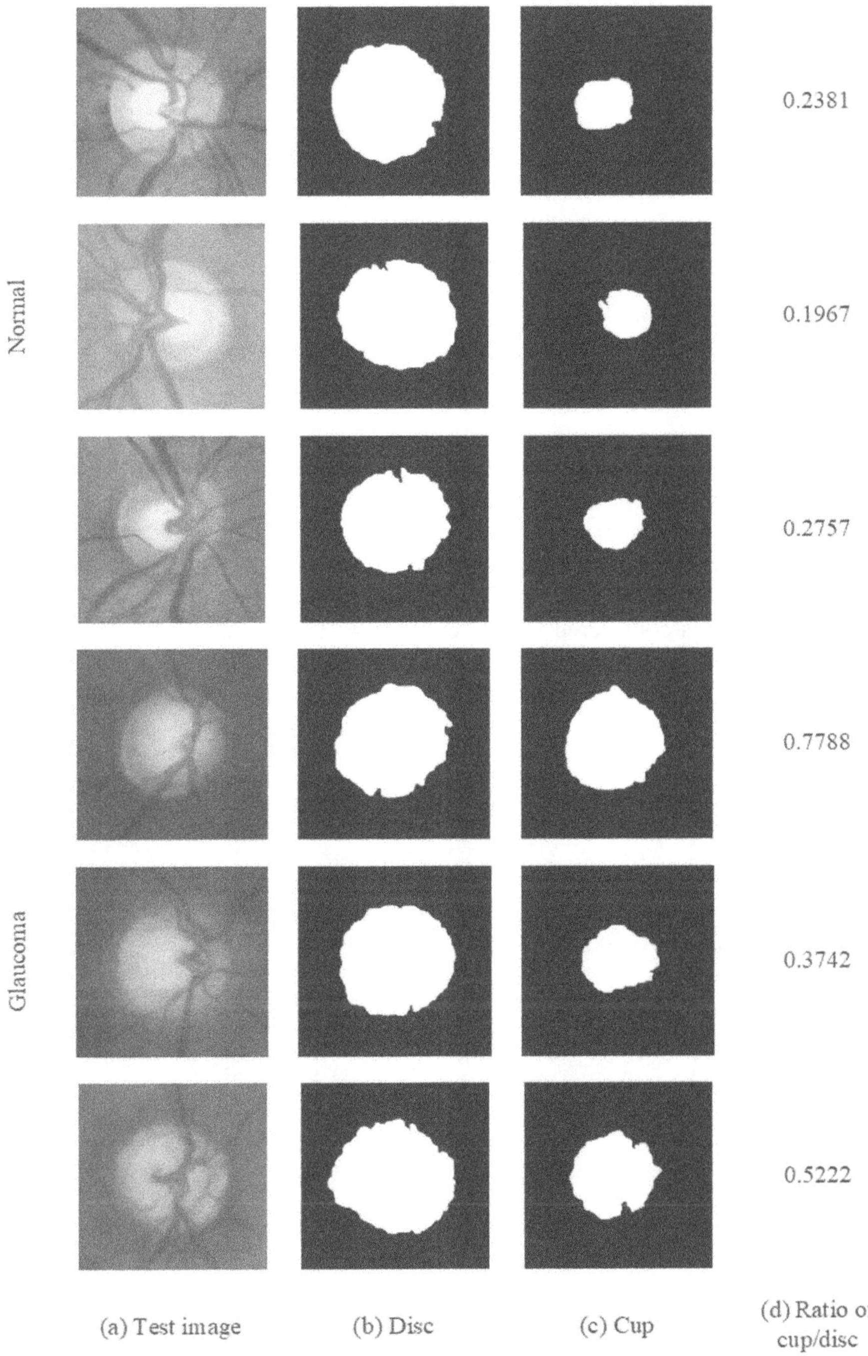

FIGURE 5.4 Examination of the fundus image to evacuate the disease

TABLE 5.2
Total Number of 2D Brain MRI Considered in the Proposed Work

Modality	Database	MRI class	Training images	Validation images
DW	ISLES2015	Benign	120	34
		Malignant	150	48
	Clinical	Benign + Malignant	5+5=10	5+5=10
Total			280	92
Flair	BRATS	Benign	90	35
	(2013 & 2015)	Malignant	200	75
	Clinical	Benign + Malignant	5+5=10	5+5=10
Total			300	120

Table 5.2 presents the total numbers of test image considered for the investigation. This table also presents the number of images considered for to train and validate the considered classifier system.

Figure 5.5 and 5.6 depicts the sample test pictures of ISLES2015 (DW modality) and BRATS 2013&2015 (Flair modality) respectively. Initially, the ISLES database of chosen was considered for the evaluation. This dataset contains the MRI acquired with different modalities, like Flair, T1 and DW, with a pixel dimension of 77x77x1. This dataset also includes GT presented by a radiologist. It is a 3D dataset

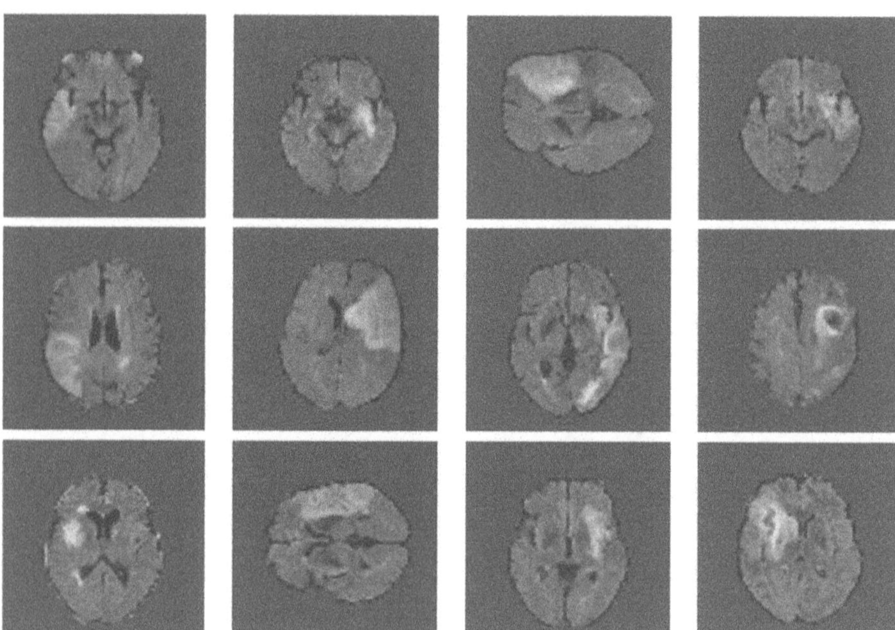

FIGURE 5.5 Sample DW modality images of ISLES2015 dataset

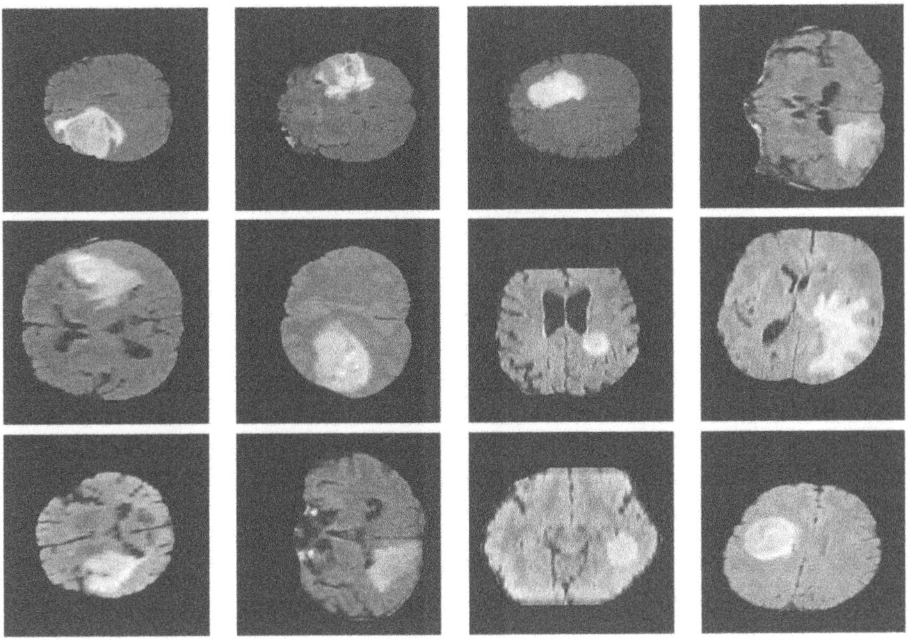

FIGURE 5.6 Sample Flair modality images of BRATS 2013 & 2015

and supports the axial, coronal and sagittal views. Initially, the chosen 2D slices from the 3D images were extracted and then re-sized into 256x256x1 pixel image. During this study, only the axial view images were considered for the evaluation.

The performance of developed image processing system is appraised with the DW and Flair modalities with various category of brain MRIs, like benign (low grade) and malignant (high grade). Initially, the proposed examination process is executed on the DW modality MRIs and the enhancement and the extraction of the tumour section is done using the chosen pre-processing and post-processing system. The ultimate aim of the system is to classify the MRI into two classes, such as healthy and the disease class.

5.3.1 Pre-processing

The pre-processing system helps to alter the available brain image into usable form. Initially, 3D to 2D conversion is implemented. Later, all the considered 2D slices are resized into 256x256x1 pixels before the image processing task.

The resized brain MRI (DW/flair modality) is then considered for the examination. Initially the abnormal section in the MRI is enhanced using the SGO and Shannon's entropy-based thresholding technique with a chosen threshold value (Th = 3). This operation helps to separate the brain image into three sections, such as abnormal region, normal brain part and the background. After the separation using the implemented thresholding task, the brain abnormality is then extracted using a chosen segmentation technique and the extracted section is then considered for the automated disease diagnosis.

5.3.2 Post-processing

The post processing operation is normally used to extract the ROI (stroke/tumour) from the test image for further assessment. In most of the machine-learning based detection system, the chosen segmentation technique is implemented as the post-processing scheme, which helps to extract the ROI with better accuracy. The post-processing methodology implemented to evaluate the brain MRI is presented below.

5.3.2.1 Active-Contour (AC)

Active contour is one of the most successful adjustable snake (line) based technique normally considered to extract the chosen regions from the medical images. In this work, the AC is to be initiated at a chosen location and is allowed to expand on the image section by discovering the identical pixels in the image section. This work also suffers due to the multi-class pixel group and yields a negative result for the uneven and poor images. The essential information on AC can be found in (Kass et al., 1988; Cohen, 1991). The convergence rate of AC is large compared to the LS and CV segmentation techniques.

5.3.2.2 Marker-Controlled-Watershed (MCWS)

The infected fragment of LGG brain image may be extorted with the semi/automated events. Semi-automated exercise requires the help of a human-operator to start the task. Hence, automatic practice is widely preferred especially for medical pictures. This work implements the Marker-Controlled-Watershed (MCWS) Mining (WS) to mine the irregular segment in MRI. MCWS involves in perimeter detection, formation of WS, modification of marker rate to mark the pixel groups, by augmenting the recognized pixels and determination of accepted region (Yang et al., 2006; Parvati et al., 2008). This MCWS helps to extort all the probable pixels from the MRI. Comparable practice is then implemented for other images.

5.3.2.3 Seed-Region-Growing (SRG)

It is one of the semi-automate segmentation procedures, in which an initiated seed grows rapidly to identify alike pixels, which has similar structure like the seeded section. The SRG works well on smooth surface and offers poor results, if the seeded area is with an un-even pixel distribution. It is one of the classical segmentation technique considered by the researchers to extract the required section from the trial image under study. The related information on SRG can be found in (Mehnert and Jackway, 1997; Tang, 2010).

5.3.3 Feature Extraction, Selection and Validation

After enhancing the considered test images using SGO assisted thresholding and a chosen segmentation technique, the essential image features are then extracted using the well-known GLCM approach (Haralick et al., 1973; Aksoy and Haralick, 1998). The GLCM is one of the commonly texture feature extraction procedure normally used in the image processing techniques to classify the considered images into various classes based on the need.

The GLCM helps to extract nearly twenty-five features from each image and the extracted features differs based on the abnormality and this difference is then considered to classify the images using a chosen classifier. If the entire features of the GLCM are implemented, the proposed system may suffer due to over fitting problem and hence, a feature reduction technique is essential to reduce the image features from 25 numbers to a lower number. The feature reduction can be implemented using statistical approaches (Student's t-test) or heuristic algorithm-based techniques. The heuristic algorithm assisted approach is quite simple compared to the traditional statistical technique. In this work, the Bat Algorithm (BA) based feature selection discussed in (Bakiya et al., 2020) is considered to find the dominant features and for the GLCM case, the proposed BA technique helped to select 10 dominant features.

The selected features are then considered to train, test and validate the classifier unit; which helps to classify the considered brain MRI slices into normal and disease classes. In the proposed work, well known common classifiers, such as Adaptive Neuro-Fuzzy Inference System (ANFIS), Decision-Tree 9DT0, Random-Forest (RF) and K-Nearest Neighbour (KNN) are considered to implement two class classifications.

Adaptive Neuro-Fuzzy Inference System

ANFIS assisted categorization is a well-recognized process to classify the medicinal data with the selected features. This system was constructed by incorporating the neural-network principle and Takagi–Sugeno fuzzy suggestion. The supposition configuration in ANFIS works based on a set of Fuzzy IF–THEN rules, which surround the learning prospective to estimate nonlinear functions. Due to its capability, ANFIS is usually used to classify medical signals and images. In this system, the ANFIS structure is implemented as follows; the training phase is realized in two stages, such as forward and reverse. During the forward training task, least square technique is implemented and during the backward training task, minimization of the overall quadratic cost value is executed. While performing these tasks, this algorithm determines the optimal set of parameters to be considered during testing process. The initial parameters of ANFIS is assigned as follows; (i) Bell-shaped membership function is adopted in the fuzzy system, (ii) Iteration number is assigned as 500, (iii) Parameter adaptation step size is chosen as 0.01 and (iv) Error acceptance was fixed as 0.001. The essential information regarding ANFIS can be found in (Güler and Übeyli, 2015; Chang and Chang, 2006; Dey et al., 2019).

Decision-Tree

DT is widely considered to categorize the linear/non-linear features with a progression of testing methods, which evolves similar to a tree-like flow diagram. It utilizes a distinctive assessment setting like the root and inner nodes, and the class label forms terminal nodes. Once a DT has been formed, classification is attained with possible conclusions reached in every distribution of the tree. Essential information regarding the DT supported classification is found in (Safavian and Landgrebe, 1991; Friedl and Brodley, 1997).

Random-Forest

RF is an enhanced practice and robust to noise and proficient on massive datasets. It designated with a set of tree predictors in which each tree is depending on a subjective vector. This vector is sampled independently like the similar allotment of trees in the dense forest region. This practice is reasonably speedy and it is straightforward in execution. RF can be mathematically represented as in Eqn. (5.1);

$$R(q) = argmax_b \sum^{K} I(h_1(T) = Y) \tag{5.1}$$

where $R(q)$ denotes the finishing mutual classifier, K signify the appraisal tree number, $h_1(x)$ explain the decision tree, class label illustrated by Y and $I(h_1(T) = Y)$ designate that the T belongs to class Y. Other information on the RF classifier is discussed in (Pal, 2005; Díaz-Uriarte and De Andres, 2006; Svetnik et al., 2003).

K-Nearest Neighbour

When the KNN is executed, it approximates the space from a sequence of novel information to all training data points, and realizes the straight point as the finest

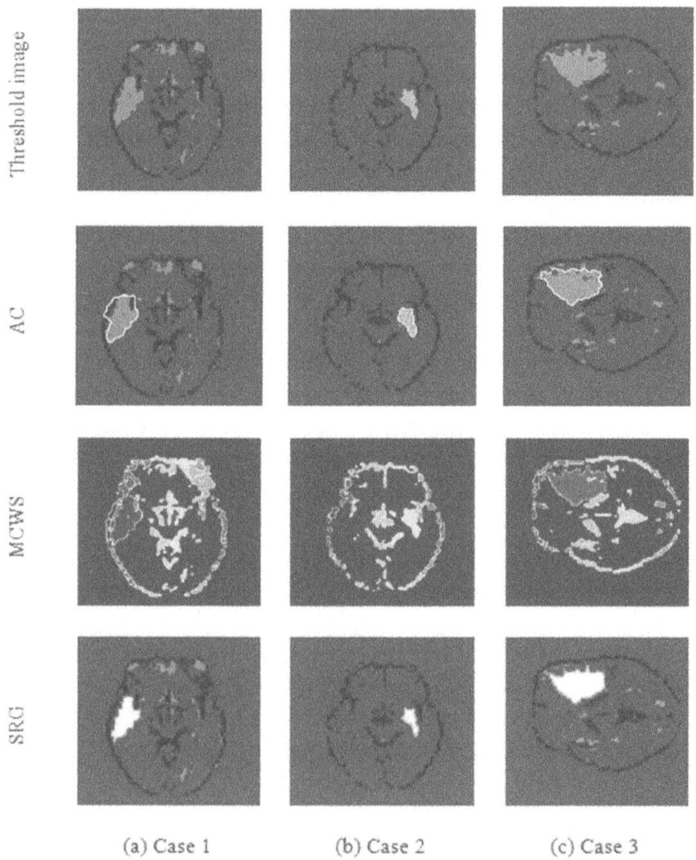

FIGURE 5.7 Sample results obtained with the DW MRI slices

neighbour. The K consequence is empirically calculated using the training sample's associated error. The mathematical form of KNN is depicted as below:

Let $X = (X_1, X_2, \ldots X_n)^T$ and $Y = (Y_1, Y_2, \ldots Y_n)^T$ demotes the two characteristic vectors of chosen magnitude with the following Euclidean distance;

$$Euclidean\ distance\ (\vec{X}, \vec{Y}) = \sqrt{(X_1 - Y_1)^2 + (X_2 - Y_2)^2 +, \ldots, +(M_D - N_1)^2} \tag{5.2}$$

Eqn. (5.2) helps to identify the distance between the vectors and based on this information, it classifies the considered information. The essential information on KNN is accessible from (Coomans and Massart, 1982; Hautamaki et al., 2004; Cunningham and Delany, 2020).

The proposed scheme is implemented separately on the ISLES and the BRATS dataset and the attained thresholding and the segmentation results are presented in Figure 5.7 and Figure 5.8 respectively. In the proposed work the Shannon's entropy thresholding helps to improve the images with better visibility and later, the abnormal

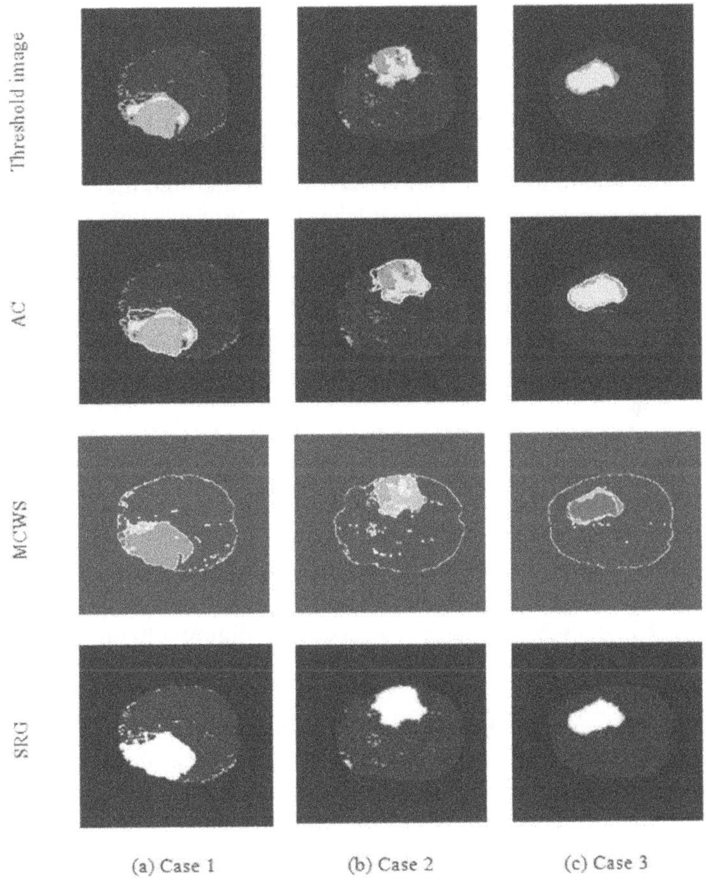

FIGURE 5.8 Sample experimental outcome obtained with flair MRI slices

TABLE 5.3
Chosen GLCM Features Using the Bat Algorithm Based Feature Selection

	DW modality		Flair modality	
Selected features	**Mean±SD (Normal)**	**Mean±SD (Stroke)**	**Mean±SD (Normal)**	**Mean±SD (Tumour)**
Autocorrelation	1.0216±0.0081	1.0128±0.0076	1.0410±0.0134	1.0453±0.0128
Cluster-prominence	0.0462±0.0097	0.0488±0.0113	0.2218±0.0528	0.2186±0.0489
Cluster-shade	0.0498±0.0195	0.0506±0.0216	0.1056±0.0103	0.1038±0.0095
Contrast	0.0013±0.0003	0.0012±0.0007	0.0033±0.0008	0.0034±0.0005
Correlation	0.8098±0.0136	0.8135±0.0118	0.9106±0.0252	0.9132±0.0241
Energy	0.9688±0.0128	0.9728±0.0134	0.9351±0.0304	0.9341±0.0294
Entropy	0.0413±0.0117	0.0407±0.0126	0.2096±0.0132	0.2105±0.0118
Homogeneity	0.9964±0.0022	0.9972±0.0019	0.9908±0.0014	0.9894±0.0107
IMC1	−0.5844±0.0794	−0.5736±0.0835	−0.8027±0.0108	−0.8042±0.0098
IMC2	0.2098±0.0508	0.2131±0.0418	0.3664±0.0291	0.3714±0.0306

section (ROI) in the enhanced image is extracted using AC, MCWS and SRG and from the extracted ROI, the essential texture features are then collected using the GLCM scheme. The total number of GLCM values are high (25 numbers) and this feature is then reduced to 10 using the BA based feature selection technique and the results are depicted in Table 5.3.

The features depicted in Table 5.3 are the dominant features of the MRI and then the considered classifiers (ANFIS, DT, RF and KNN) are trained and validated using this system. The proposed system is separately tested using the considered classifiers using the ISLES and the BRATS database and the attained results are presented for the confirmation.

Figures 5.9 and 5.10 depict the confusion matrix obtained for the chosen test images. In DW modality case, a sum of 372 (164 benign and 208 malignant case) images was considered for the examination. Figure 5.9 (a) presents the confusion matrix value for the ANFIS classifier with attained TP, TN, FP and FN values. These values are then considered to compute the performance measures, such as Accuracy, Precision, Sensitivity and Specificity. Figure 5.9 (b) to (d) depicts the confusion matrix of DT, RF and KNN classifiers respectively. Figure 5.10 (a) to (d) presents the confusion matrix obtained for the BRATS database with ANFIS, DT, RF and KNN classifiers respectively.

The results attained with the proposed study confirms that, the ANFIS and KNN classifier presents better result for the ISLES database (accuracy 97.04%) and the ANFIS classifier helped to achieve an accuracy of 96.67% with the BRATS database. The results attained with the brain MRI database confirms that, proposed system works is very efficient in detecting the brain abnormality using the chosen MRI images and in future, this system can be used to evaluate the clinical grade brain MRI slices.

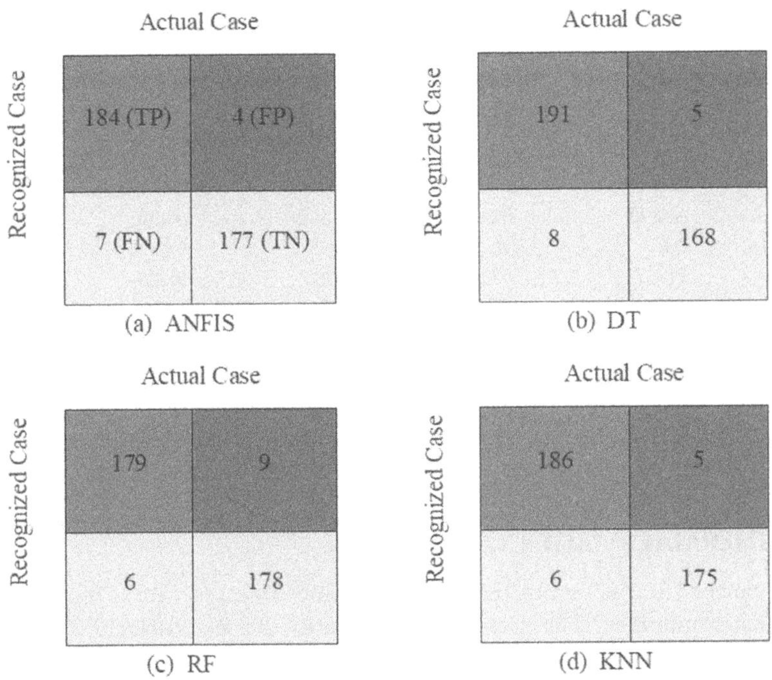

FIGURE 5.9 Confusion matrix for DW modality MRI slices

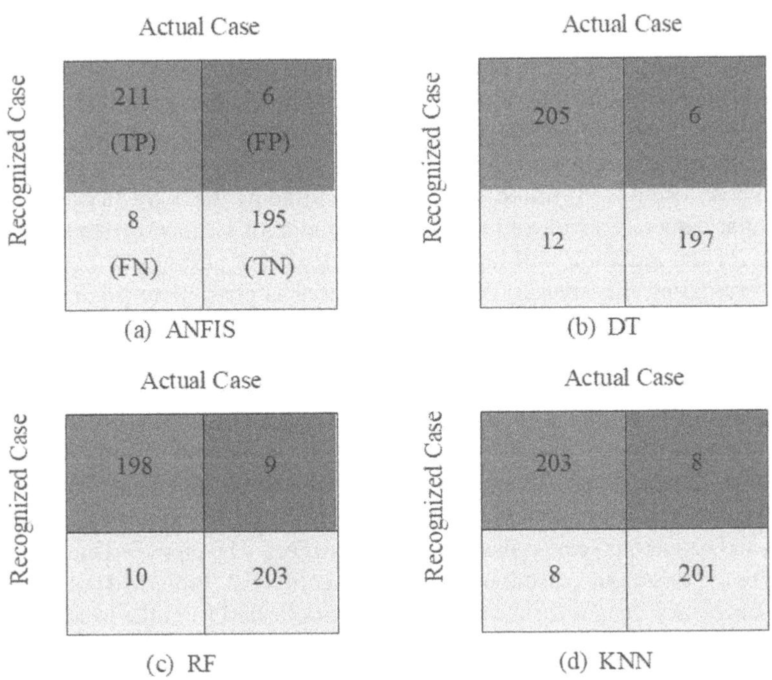

FIGURE 5.10 Confusion matrix for flair modality MRI slices

TABLE 5.4
Performance Measures Obtained With the Implemented Classifier Systems

		Performance measures (%)			
Modality	**Classifier**	**Accuracy**	**Precision**	**Sensitivity**	**Specificity**
DW	ANFIS	97.04	97.87	96.33	97.79
	DT	96.50	97.45	95.98	97.11
	RF	95.97	95.21	96.76	95.19
	KNN	97.04	97.38	96.88	97.22
Flair	ANFIS	96.67	97.24	96.35	97.01
	DT	95.71	97.16	94.47	97.04
	RF	95.48	95.65	95.19	95.75
	KNN	96.19	96.21	96.21	96.17

5.4 THERMAL IMAGE EXAMINATION

Breast cancer (BC) is one of the life-threatening illnesses with a high death rate in women comminute. The present declaration by the World-Health-Organization (WHO) verifies that breast and lung cancer is the leading cause of death compared to other cancers, and in 2018 alone a registered death rate of 2.09 million is reached. The BC affects mainly the women and in recent years, substantial awareness camps are conducted globally to reduce the occurrence rate of BC. The premature stage analysis of BC will be prepared with an individual check followed by a clinical assessment by an experienced doctor. At the clinical level, the BC can be examined and confirmed with the help of medical imaging procedures recorded with a range of modalities, such as mammograms, CT, MRI, ultrasound and thermal imaging. Thermal imaging is a newly adopted modality in clinics to identify the disease in internal body using the Infrared Waves (IW) emitted by the body. In this procedure, a particular camera is employed to capture the radiation emitted by the body and the intensity of the radiation will hold vital information regarding the body parts. By simply evaluating the intensity level in images, it is possible to predict the abnormality in the breast (Raja et al., 2017; Rajinikanth et al., 2017; Nair et al., 2018; Fernandes et al., 2019; Thanaraj et al., 2020).

The image examination system proposed to detect the BC using the thermal imaging is depicted in Figure 5.11 and the various stages clearly depicts the important operations to be implemented to detect the breast abnormality using the proposed image processing scheme. When the proposed scheme is implemented on the chosen thermal images, it is possible to classify the considered thermal image dataset into normal and cancerous section using chosen classifiers. The proposed methodology is similar to the techniques discussed in the sub-section 5.3 (brain MRI classification).

The necessary images for the assessment are collected from the benchmark database and the clinic. The information regarding the considered data can be found in the earlier research works and in the proposed scheme, the aim is to implement a

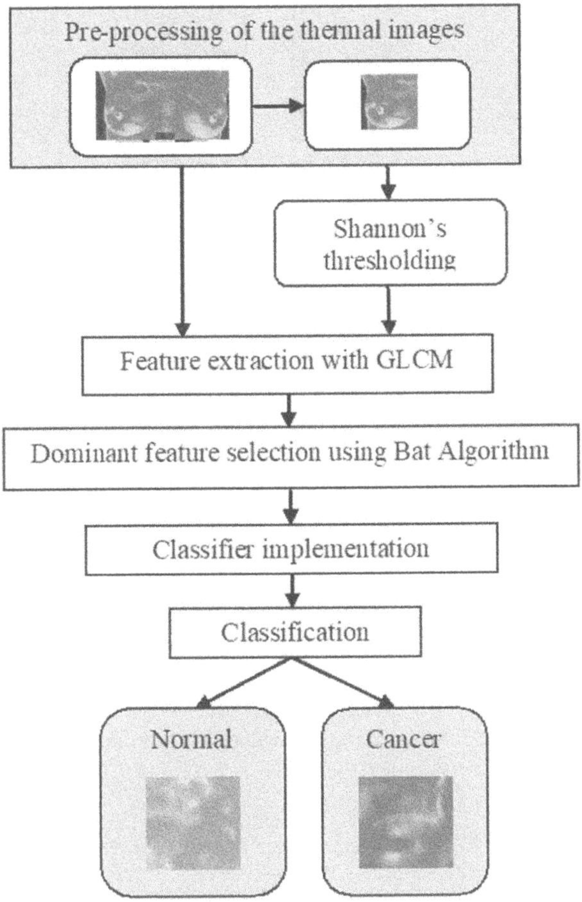

FIGURE 5.11 Block diagram, of the image processing system considered to detect the breast abnormality

classifier to classify the database into two classes (normal/cancer class). This sub-section presents the information regarding the data collection, initial data treatment and resizing operations and the other image processing operations, such as the pre-processing, post-processing, feature extraction, feature selection, classification and validation can be implemented as discussed in sub-section 5.3 (brain MRI assessment using ISLES and BRATS database).

Figure 5.13 depicts the initial level processing implemented to examine the breast abnormality. In this work, the necessary breast section is initially extracted (Figure 5.12 (a)) and then separated into two sections, such as right (Figure 5.12 (b)) and left (Figure 5.12 (c)). The separation helps to detect the asymmetry based on the size difference between the left and the right sections. The literature confirms that the infected section of the breast will have the bigger size compared to the

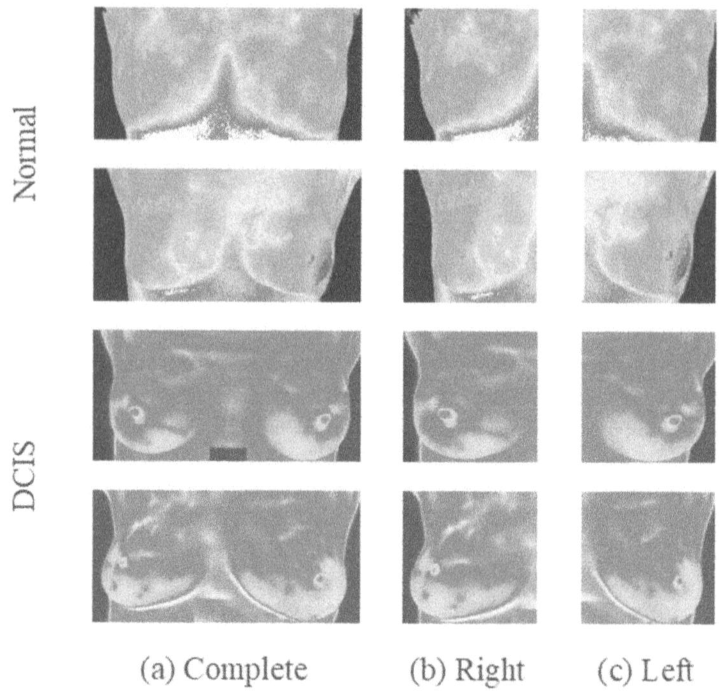

FIGURE 5.12 Initial level image processing involves in the cropping and resizing operations

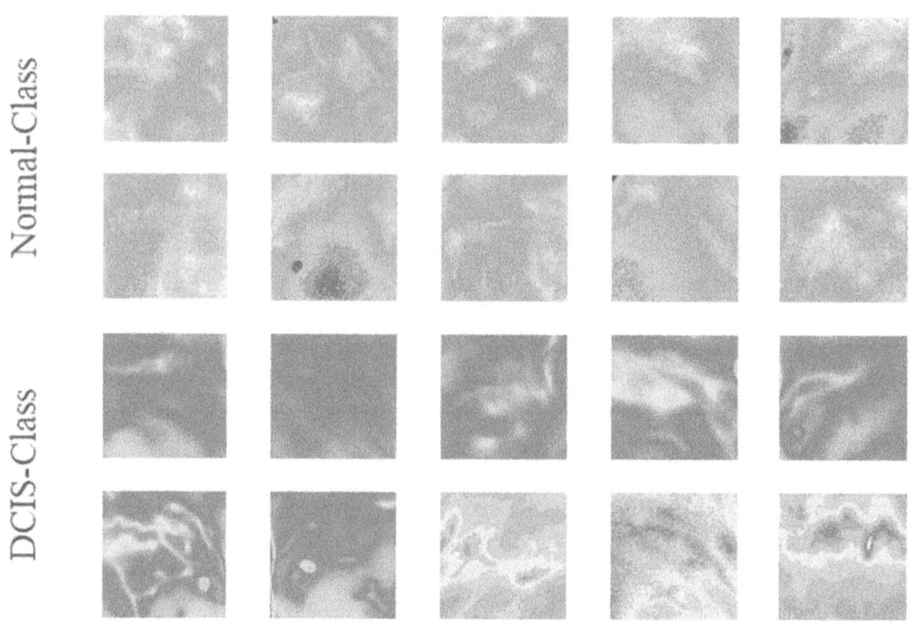

FIGURE 5.13 Abnormal section selection and resizing to implement the proposed system

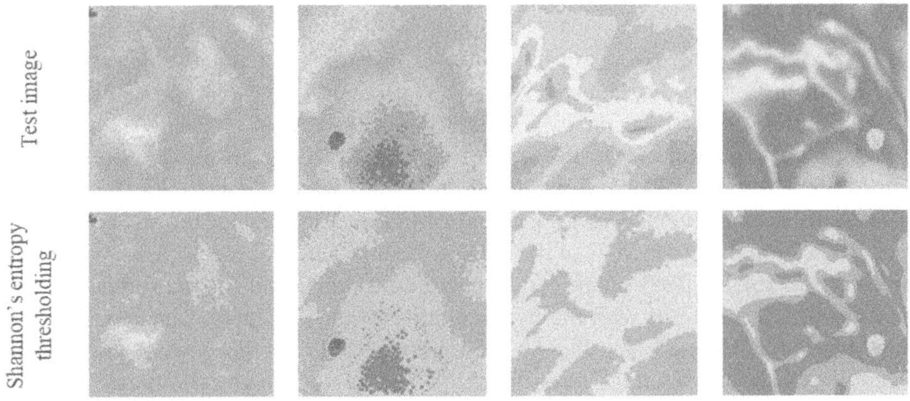

FIGURE 5.14 Original and pre-processed image using SGO and Shannon's entropy

normal breast. Hence, the initial evaluation of the asymmetry helps to verify the abnormality in the breast. Later, the infection section with various colours (bright colours, such as white, orange, pink and red) are extracted and resized into an image with dimension 256x256x3 pixels. Similar procedure is implemented on the normal breast section with green and blue colour sections and the resized images are presented in Figure 5.13 for both the normal and the abnormal (DCIS - Ductal Carcinoma In Situ) cases. The resized breast sections are pre-processed using the entropy based approaches and the essential features are then extracted using the GLCM technique. The extracted features are then reduced using Bat Algorithm and the reduced feature sub-set is finally considered to train, test and validate the classifiers, such as DT, RF and KNN. In this work, 300 images of each case is considered for the assessment and 100 images are considered to validate the performance of the classifiers. The experimental result of this study is depicted in Figure 5.14 and Table 5.5. From this table, it is verified that, the KNN classifier helped to achieve a better result (accuracy of 92%) compared to the DT (88.50%) and RF (91.50%). The results of the proposed technique confirms that, proposed technique works well on the considered thermal images and helps to detect the DCIS with better accuracy.

TABLE 5.5
Classification Results Attained With the Considered Breast Thermal Images

Classifier	TP	FN	TN	FP	Accuracy	Precision	Sensitivity	Specificity
DT	87	13	90	10	88.50	89.69	87.00	89.00
RF	92	8	91	9	91.50	91.08	92.00	91.00
KNN	94	6	90	10	92.00	90.38	94.00	90.00

5.5 SUMMARY

This part of the book discussed the image examination and disease detection procedures using a class of image modalities available in the greyscale and the RGB scales. Initial section presented the evaluation of the retinal abnormality using the FRI of a chosen database. In this work the RIM-ONE database is considered and based on the ratio of the cup/disc value the retinal illness is confirmed. The second case-study is implemented using the brain MRI slices to detect the stroke and the tumour section using the MRI of the chosen modality. For the stroke assessment, the well-known ISLES 2015 dataset images are considered and for the tumour detection the BRATS dataset with the flair modality MRI is adopted. The experimental investigation confirmed that, the ANFIS classifier helped to get better classification accuracy on both the image cases. Finally, a case-study using the breast thermal imaging is presented using the benchmark as well as the clinical grade images and the proposed technique helped to achieve better result with the KNN classifier. The experimental investigation confirmed that, when the considered medical images are pre-processed using the Shannon's entropy-based thresholding process, and then a superior result can be achieved irrespective of the image modality. This result of this section confirms the superiority of the entropy-based approaches in the medical image processing domain.

REFERENCES

Aksoy, S., & Haralick, R. M. (1998, June). Textural features for image database retrieval. In *Proceedings. IEEE Workshop on Content-Based Access of Image and Video Libraries (Cat. No. 98EX173)* (pp. 45–49). IEEE.

Bakiya, A., Kamalanand, K., Rajinikanth, V., Nayak, R. S., & Kadry, S. (2020). Deep neural network assisted diagnosis of time-frequency transformed electromyograms. *Multimedia Tools and Applications*, 79(15), 11051–11067.

Balan, N. S., Kumar, A. S., Raja, N. S. M., & Rajinikanth, V. (2016). Optimal multilevel image thresholding to improve the visibility of Plasmodium sp. in blood smear images. *Advances in Intelligent Systems and Computing*, *397*, 563–571.

Bhandary, A., Prabhu, G. A., Rajinikanth, V., Thanaraj, K. P., Satapathy, S. C., Robbins, D. E., Shasky, C., Zhang, Y. D., Tavares, J. M. R. S., & Raja, N. S. M. (2020). Deep-learning framework to detect lung abnormality–A study with chest X-Ray and lung CT scan images. *Pattern Recognition Letters*, *129*, 271–278.

Bock, R., Meier, J., Nyúl, L. G., Hornegger, J., & Michelson, G. (2010). Glaucoma risk index: automated glaucoma detection from color fundus images. *Medical image analysis*, 14(3), 471–481.

Chaki, J., & Dey, N. (2020). Data tagging in medical images: A survey of the state-of-art. *Current Medical Imaging.*

Chang, F. J., & Chang, Y. T. (2006). Adaptive neuro-fuzzy inference system for prediction of water level in reservoir. *Advances in water resources*, *29*(1), 1–10.

Cohen, L. D. (1991). On active contour models and balloons. *CVGIP: Image Understanding*, 53(2), 211–218.

Cohen, L. D. (1991). On active contour models and balloons. *CVGIP: Image understanding*, 53(2), 211–218.

Coomans, D., & Massart, D. L. (1982). Alternative k-nearest neighbour rules in supervised pattern recognition: Part 1. k-nearest neighbour classification by using alternative voting rules. *Analytica Chimica Acta, 136*, 15–27.

Cunningham, P., & Delany, S. J. (2020). k-nearest neighbour classifiers. *arXiv preprint arXiv:2004.04523.*

Dey, N., Fuqian Shi, F., & Rajinikanth, V. (2019). Leukocyte Nuclei Segmentation Using Entropy Function and Chan-Vese Approach. *Information Technology and Intelligent Transportation Systems, 314*, 255–264.

Dey, N., Rajinikanth, V., Shi, F., Tavares, J. M. R., Moraru, L., Karthik, K. A., & Emmanuel, C. (2019). Social-Group-Optimization based tumor evaluation tool for clinical brain MRI of Flair/diffusion-weighted modality. *Biocybernetics and Biomedical Engineering*, 39(3), 843–856.

Dey, N., Shi, F., & Rajinikanth, V. (2020). Image examination system to detect gastric polyps from endoscopy images. *Information Technology and Intelligent Transportation Systems*, 323, 107–116.

Díaz-Uriarte, R., & De Andres, S. A. (2006). Gene selection and classification of microarray data using random forest. *BMC Bioinformatics*, 7(1), 3.

Dvořák, P., & Menze, B. (2015). Local structure prediction with convolutional neural networks for multimodal brain tumor segmentation. In *International MICCAI Workshop on Medical Computer Vision* (pp. 59). Springer.

Fernandes, S. L., Rajinikanth, V., & Kadry, S. (2019). A hybrid framework to evaluate breast abnormality using infrared thermal images. *IEEE Consumer Electronics Magazine*, 8(5), 31–36.

Fernandes, S. L., Rajinikanth, V., & Kadry, S. (2019). A hybrid framework to evaluate breast abnormality using infrared thermal images. *IEEE Consumer Electronics Magazine*, 8(5), 31–36.

Friedl, M. A., & Brodley, C. E. (1997). Decision tree classification of land cover from remotely sensed data. *Remote Sensing of Environment*, 61(3), 399–409.

Fumero, F., Alayón, S., Sanchez, J. L., Sigut, J., & Gonzalez-Hernandez, M. (2011, June). RIM-ONE: an open retinal image database for optic nerve evaluation. In *2011 24th international symposium on computer-based medical systems (CBMS)* (pp. 1–6). IEEE.

Güler, I., & Übeyli, E. D. (2005). Adaptive neuro-fuzzy inference system for classification of EEG signals using wavelet coefficients. *Journal of Neuroscience Methods*, 148(2), 113–121.

Haralick, R. M., Shanmugam, K., & Dinstein, I. H. (1973). Textural features for image classification. *IEEE Transactions on systems, man, and cybernetics*, (6), 610–621.

Hautamaki, V., Karkkainen, I., & Franti, P. (2004). Outlier detection using k-nearest neighbour graph. In *Proceedings of the 17th International Conference on Pattern Recognition, 2004. ICPR 2004.* (Vol. 3, pp. 430–433). IEEE.

http://www.cdc.gov/dpdx/trypanosomiasisAmerican/gallery.html. (Accessed on: 15 March 2020).

https://uwaterloo.ca/vision-image-processing-lab/research-demos/skin-cancer-detection. (Accessed on: 15 March 2020).

Jesline, R., Francelin, A. J. T., & Rajinikanth, V. S., V. (2020). Development of a semiautomated evaluation procedure for dermoscopy pictures with hair segment. *Advances in Intelligent Systems and Computing*, 1119. 283–292.

Kass, M., Witkin, A., & Terzopoulos, D. (1988). Snakes: active contour models. *International Journal of Computer Vision*, 1(4), 321–331.

Kass, M., Witkin, A., &Terzopoulos, D. (1988). Snakes: Active contour models. *International Journal of Computer Vision*, 1(4), 321–331.

Lakshmi, V. S., Tebby, S. G., Shriranjani, D., & Rajinikanth, V. (2016). Chaotic cuckoo search and Kapur/Tsallis approach in segmentation of T. Cruzi from blood smear images. *International Journal of Computer Science and Information Security (IJCSIS)*, 14(CIC 2016), 51–56.

Li, C., Xu, C., Gui, C., & Fox, M. D. (2005). Level set evolution without re-initialization: a new variational formulation. In 2005 IEEE computer society conference on computer vision and pattern recognition (CVPR'05) (Vol. 1, pp. 430–436). IEEE.

Liu, J., Wong, D. W. K., Lim, J. H., Li, H., Tan, N. M., & Wong, T. Y. (2009). ARGALI: an automatic cup-to-disc ratio measurement system for glaucoma detection and AnaLysIs framework. In *Medical Imaging 2009: Computer-Aided Diagnosis* (Vol. 7260, p. 72603K). International Society for Optics and Photonics.

Maier, O., Menze, B. H., von der Gablentz, J., Häni, L., Heinrich, M. P., Liebrand, M., & Christiaens, D. (2017). ISLES 2015-a public evaluation benchmark for ischemic stroke lesion segmentation from multispectral MRI. *Medical image analysis*, *35*, 250–269.

Maier, O., Wilms, M., & Handels, H. (2015). Image features for brain lesion segmentation using random forests. In *BrainLes 2015* (pp. 119). Springer.

Manickavasagam, K., Sutha, S., & Kamalanand, K. (2014). An automated system based on 2d empirical mode decomposition and k-means clustering for classification of Plasmodium species in thin blood smear images. *BMC Infect Dis.*, 14(Suppl 3), P13.

Mehnert, A., & Jackway, P. (1997). An improved seeded region growing algorithm. *Pattern Recognition Letters*, 18(10), 1065–1071.

Mehnert, A., & Jackway, P. (1997). An improved seeded region growing algorithm. *Pattern Recognition Letters*, 18(10), 1065–1071.

Menze, B. H., Jakab, A., Bauer, S., Kalpathy-Cramer, J., Farahani, K., Kirby, J., & Lanczi, L. (2014). The multimodal brain tumor image segmentation benchmark (BRATS). *IEEE Transactions on Medical Imaging*, 34(10), 1993–2024.

Menze, B., Jakab, A., Bauer, S., Reyes, M., Prastawa, M., & Van Leemput, K. (2012). Proceedings of the miccai challenge on multimodal brain tumor image segmentation (brats) 2012

Nair, M. V., Gnanaprakasam, C. N., Rakshana, R., Keerthana, N., & Rajinikanth, V. (2018). Investigation of breast melanoma using hybrid image-processing-tool. In *2018 International Conference on Recent Trends in Advance Computing (ICRTAC)* (pp. 174–179). IEEE.

Nguyen, H. T., Worring, M., & Van Den Boomgaard, R. (2003). Watersnakes: energy-driven watershed segmentation. *IEEE Transactions on Pattern Analysis and Machine Intelligence*, 25(3), 330–342.

Pal, M. (2005). Random forest classifier for remote sensing classification. *International Journal of Remote Sensing*, 26(1), 217–222.

Parvati, K., Rao, P., & Mariya Das, M. (2008). Image segmentation using gray-scale morphology and marker-controlled watershed transformation. *Discrete Dynamics in Nature and Society.*

Raja, N. S. M., Rajinikanth, V., Fernandes, S. L., & Satapathy, S. C. (2017). Segmentation of breast thermal images using Kapur's entropy and hidden Markov random field. *Journal of Medical Imaging and Health Informatics*, 7(8), 1825–1829.

Raja, N., Rajinikanth, V., Fernandes, S. L., & Satapathy, S. C. (2017). Segmentation of breast thermal images using Kapur's entropy and hidden Markov random field. *Journal of Medical Imaging and Health Informatics*, 7(8), 1825–1829.

Rajinikanth, V., Raja, N. S. M., & Arunmozhi, S. (2019). ABCD rule implementation for the skin melanoma assessment–a study, In. IEEE International Conference on System, Computation, Automation and Networking (ICSCAN), 1–4. IEEE.

Rajinikanth, V., Raja, N. S. M., Satapathy, S. C., Dey, N., & Devadhas, G. G. (2017). Thermogram assisted detection and analysis of ductal carcinoma in situ (DCIS). In *2017 International Conference on Intelligent Computing, Instrumentation and Control Technologies (ICICICT)* (pp. 1641–1646). IEEE.

Rajinikanth,V., Dey, N., Kavallieratou, E., & Lin, H. (2020) Firefly Algorithm-Based Kapur's Thresholding and Hough Transform to Extract Leukocyte Section from Hematological Images. In: Dey, N. (eds) Applications of Firefly Algorithm and its Variants. *Springer Tracts in Nature-Inspired Computing*, 221–235. Springer.

Rezatofighi, S. H., & Soltanian-Zadeh, H. (2011). Automatic recognition of five types of white blood cells in peripheral blood. *Comput Med Imaging Graph*, 35(4), 333–343.

Safavian, S. R., & Landgrebe, D. (1991). A survey of decision tree classifier methodology. *IEEE Transactions on Systems, Man, and Cybernetics*, 21(3), 660–674.

Shafarenko, L., Petrou, M., & Kittler, J. (1997). Automatic watershed segmentation of randomly textured color images. *IEEE transactions on Image Processing*, 6(11), 1530–1544.

Sharma, P., Sample, P. A., Zangwill, L. M., & Schuman, J. S. (2008). Diagnostic tools for glaucoma detection and management. *Survey of ophthalmology*, 53(6), S17–S32.

Sivaswamy, J., Krishnadas, S., Chakravarty, A., Joshi, G., & Tabish, A. S. (2015). A comprehensive retinal image dataset for the assessment of glaucoma from the optic nerve head analysis. *JSM Biomedical Imaging Data Papers*, 2(1), 1004.

Svetnik, V., Liaw, A., Tong, C., Culberson, J. C., Sheridan, R. P., & Feuston, B. P. (2003). Random forest: a classification and regression tool for compound classification and QSAR modeling. *Journal of Chemical Information and Computer Sciences*, 43(6), 1947–1958.

Tang, J. (2010). A color image segmentation algorithm based on region growing. In *2010 2nd International Conference on Computer Engineering and Technology* (Vol. 6, pp. V6–634). IEEE.

Thanaraj, R. I. R., Anand, B., Rahul, J. A., & Rajinikanth, V. (2020). Appraisal of Breast Ultrasound Image Using Shannon's Thresholding and Level-Set Segmentation. In *Progress in Computing, Analytics and Networking* (pp. 621). Springer.

Xu, W., & Cumming, I. (1999). A region-growing algorithm for InSAR phase unwrapping. *IEEE Transactions on Geoscience and Remote Sensing*, 37(1), 124–134.

Yang, X., Li, H., & Zhou, X. (2006). Nuclei segmentation using marker-controlled watershed, tracking using mean-shift, and Kalman filter in time-lapse microscopy. *IEEE Transactions on Circuits and Systems I: Regular Papers*, 53(11), 2405–2414.

Yu, S., Xiao, D., Frost, S., & Kanagasingam, Y. (2019). Robust optic disc and cup segmentation with deep learning for glaucoma detection. *Computerized Medical Imaging and Graphics*, *74*, 61–71.

Index

S

T

U

V

For Product Safety Concerns and Information please contact our EU
representative GPSR@taylorandfrancis.com
Taylor & Francis Verlag GmbH, Kaufingerstraße 24, 80331 München, Germany

www.ingramcontent.com/pod-product-compliance
Ingram Content Group UK Ltd.
Pitfield, Milton Keynes, MK11 3LW, UK
UKHW020207200926
475702UK00004B/659
* 9 7 8 0 3 6 7 4 7 3 9 4 5 *